San Francisco Coroner's Office:

A History 1850-1980

San Francisco Coroner's Office:

A History 1850-1980

by

Terence Beckington Allen MD

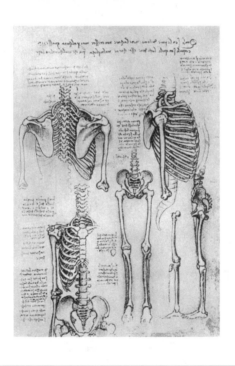

Redactors' Press
San Francisco California

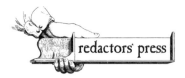

David and Sallie Allen
1400 Geary Blvd, Suite 115 • San Francisco CA 94109-6561
voice phone 415/929-0253 • *fax phone* 415/567-2576
email. sarahple@ix.netcom.com

© 2002 1999 by Terence Beckington Allen
Jacket, interior design, & production: Phillip Dizick

No part of this publication may be reproduced or transmitted
in any form or by any means electronic or mechanical, including
photocopy, recording, or any information storage and retrieval
system now known or to be invented, without permission in
writing from the publisher, except by a receiver or reader who
wishes to quote brief passages in connection with a review
written for inclusion in a magazine, newspaper, or broadcast.

Publisher's Cataloging-in-Publication
(Provided by Quality Books, Inc.)

Allen, Terence, 1950-
    San Francisco coroner's office : a history 1850-1980
/by Terence, Beckington Allen. —3rd ed.
    p. cm.
    Includes bibliographical references and index.
    LCCN: 2002102461
    ISBN: 0-9718328-0-3

    1. San Francisco (Calif.). Coroner—History.
2. Forensic pathology—California—San Francisco—History.
3. Coroners—California—San Francisco—History.
4. Medical examiners (Law)—California—San Francisco—
History. I. Title.

RA1063.4.A45 2002   614'.1'0979461
                QB102-200073

Printed in the United States of America
3rd edition [revised 1999]

for
Kim Marie Thorburn

Terence Beckington Allen MD, certified as an anatomic and forensic pathologist by the American Board of Pathology, wrote this history of the San Francisco Medical Examiner-Coroner's Office during the period he was working there as a forensic pathology resident-in-training or as an assistant medical examiner (1977-82). He is at the time of this edition a general physician on the staff of Eastern State Hospital, Medical Lake, Washington. Allen is married to Kim Marie Thorburn MD, Public Health Officer, Spokane Region, Washington State.

Terence Beckington Allen MD
West 8121 Rutter Pkwy
Spokane WA 99208-9244

Voice phone 509/465-3025
Fax phone 509/465-4695
Email kthorburn@msn.com

Contents

Preface and acknowledgements

This book was published in serial form in *San Francisco Medicine* 1982-83. Before that there was an edition printed in manuscript form and presented to the University of California San Francisco (UCSF) Library while the author was a resident in forensic pathology.

The author earlier interviewed many individuals. Staffs of San Francisco Main Library, University of California San Francisco Library, University of California Hastings Law School Library, California Historical Society in San Francisco, and the San Francisco City Morgue gave time and assistance for information and references.

The author gave permission to David Walton Allen and Sarah Peelle Allen to reprint this third edition as a more complete history with cited references that had not before been published. Quotations have been changed only to fit the style and format of numerals used for this publication. The style manual used is the 1994 *New York Public Library Writer's Guide to Style and Usage First Edition,* particularly in the treatment of numbers.

The publisher thanks Bill Wright as a reader, Stone Allen for library work, and Sarah Dizick for some of the original source work in San Francisco libraries.

David Allen and Sallie Allen
The Sequoias-San Francisco
June 2002

Introduction

The history of life in San Francisco is a subject for many authors, but few have considered the history of death in this city. For over 130 years a single institution, the San Francisco Coroner's Office, has objectively observed the phenomena of sudden or unexpected deaths. Coroners and their deputies have penetrated the streets at all hours to peer into squalid sick beds and dark alleys, seeing the effects of violence and catastrophe. The work of the coroner and his agents is not always pleasant but always human. A history of San Francisco Coroners' work is one history of the City. My writing here is specifically a history of the San Francisco Coroner's Office collected from books, municipal records, newspapers, medical journals, and medical society proceedings. I want to portray the character of the people who held the office of the San Francisco Coroner. You can glimpse their intentions, campaigns, comments, and contributions.

Throughout this writing I shall pay particular attention to the development of coroners' three powers: 1) the power to investigate; 2) the power to conduct autopsies; and 3) the power to hold an inquest or judicial inquiry before a jury. In this way you can understand—as a punster put it—the "coronerstone" of the present San Francisco Coroner's Office.

Using both the *Oxford English Dictionary* and the American unabridged *Random House Dictionary of the English Language,* the word coroner comes from *coronae* meaning guardian of the pleas of the crown. The *coronator* in the *Magna Carta* was charged with "maintaining the rights of the private property of the crown.... In modern times his [coroner's] chief function is to hold inquest on the bodies of those supposed to have died by violence or accident, hence a coroner's 12 jurymen or a coroner's inquest." By usage the modern first meaning of inquest is "usually before a jury, especially in the cause of a death."

As an example, in 1800s San Francisco, colorful characters such as Joshua A Norton, "Emperor Norton I," the self-styled "Emperor of North America and Protector of Mexico," wound up in a Coroner's investigation. The Coroner's deputy was called to the scene one 1880 January day when Norton collapsed and died on California Street near the earlier St. Mary's Cathedral. The Coroner's agent took charge of the person and possessions of this popularly known figure, and these remains were delivered by horse-drawn wagon to the City Morgue. An autopsy by police surgeons showed sanguineous apoplexy, in modern terms a cerebrovascular hemorrhage. A deputy then went to investigate Norton's lodging at 624 Commercial Street. The municipal records tell us that the Emperor's possessions—including five canes, an umbrella, and a sabre—were delivered to the California Society of Pioneers in San Francisco. [1,2]

The Coroner's Office of San Francisco City and County has been a forerunner for coroners' systems in California, setting early standards. By 1900 the Office already had written reports of over 20,000 deaths. And deputies or agents had performed over 9000 autopsy procedures and reported on 994 murders, 2839 suicides, and 4222 accidental deaths. [3]

The San Francisco Coroner advocated scientific analysis from early times. By the late 1800s the autopsy rate was well over 90 percent of all cases considered sudden or unexpected deaths. Forensic documentation developed early, including toxicology, microscopy, and photography. The 30 Coroners of San Francisco have all been physicians except for the first 4, and, later, perhaps, the infamous Charles C O'Donnell who during 1885-87 passed himself off successfully, at first at least, as a physician.

The medical community supported the medical importance of the Coroner's Office, and some of San Francisco's foremost physicians were Coroners. Coroners' names like R Beverly Cole MD, a dean of Toland Medical School, and Jonathan Letterman MD, a medical director of the Army of the Republic, are familiar to those acquainted with the history of medicine in San Francisco.

In 1867 San Francisco Health Officer I Rowell MD said

> ...it is more easy to satisfy mankind of the value of any other branch of statistics than that which relates to the number that die annually, their ages, sex, occupation, condition, and nativity, and the causes which produce such deaths....[4]

A laudatory 1931 description would fit almost any year since 1850.

> Recommendations by the Coroner and his juries have led to passage of safety laws and ordinances[,] and innumerable lives of workmen and others have been saved as a result.... The generally excellent standard of the Coroner's Office in San Francisco is one of which its citizens may indeed be proud.

Yet, the general public usually has little interest in the routine function of the Coroner's Office, outside of a certain morbid curiosity or the dedicated fascination of certain news agencies. The public eye falls on the coroner only in the most dire events, and his daily work goes unnoticed. Some people seem to feel that because the Coroner deals only with the dead his work does not affect the living.[5]

In his 1979 annual report letter, Coroner Boyd G Stephens MD said

The public concept of death, along with its fears and misconceptions, is changing slowly. However, most people do not understand what we do and would really not wish to find out—until they have a family tragedy in which we have to answer to the courts or the family as to the cause and manner of death. Only at that time do they begin to realize our function and impact on the state of the community.[6]

The recipient of that letter, San Francisco Mayor George Moscone, tragically himself came under the Coroner's jurisdiction after assassination by then County Board Supervisor Dan White.

San Francisco Coroners and their Autopsy Surgeons

Coroners according to beginning year*	Autopsy Surgeons**
1850 E Gallagher	
1851 N Gray	
1853 J W Whaling	
1855 J H Kent	
1857 J M McNulty MD	
1862 B A Sheldon MD	
1865 S R Harris MD	
1868 Jonathan Letterman MD	
1872 J D B Stillman MD	Edwin Bently MD
1874 John R Rice MD	
1874 Benjamin R Swan MD	John T Crook MD
1878 Levi L Dorr MD	Drs [sic] Blach, Clarke
1882 F L Weeks MD	Drs Blach, Stambaugh
1883 Marc Levingston MD	Drs Blach, Dennis
1885 Charles Carroll O'Donnell MD	Drs Blach, Dennis
1887 James Stanton MD ˙	Dr Blach
1889 William E Taylor MD	
1891 William T Garwood MD	
1893 Jerome Hughes MD	Dr O'Connell
1895 W J Hawkins MD	George B Sommers MD
1898 Edward E Hill MD	
1899 R Beverly Cole MD	Thomas B W Leland MD
1901 Thomas B W Leland MD	Ostroilo S Kucich MD
1906 William J Walsh MD	
1908 Thomas B W Leland MD	John R Clark MD
1910 William J Walsh MD	
1911 J M Toner MD	
1912 Thomas B W Leland MD	Irving Walsh MD
	L D Bacigalupi MD
	Zera Bolin MD
	A J Remmel MD
	M E Maguns MD
	Attilus Gianini MD
	C A Glaser MD
	Sherman Leland MD
	Rolla B Hess MD
	Jesse L Carr MD
	A M Moody MD
	A Berger MD
1941 John Kingston MD	
1951 Henry W Turkel MD	
1971- Boyd G Stephens MD	

*as stated in varied municipal and country records.
**Autopsy surgeons perhaps numbered too many to list them separately in all
City and County records, and those listed did not always include a first name.

San Francisco Coroner's Office:

A History 1850-1980

1

What does a coroner do?

In California a coroner is a peace officer who investigates and documents the circumstances surrounding deaths which may not be natural or which may affect the community-at-large.

California law specifies which deaths must be reported to a coroner, and how a coroner acts in these cases. A coroner is *not* everywhere in California a physician. In most California counties the office of coroner is combined with another public office such as sheriff, district attorney, or public administrator. Usually a California coroner is an elected official, but in some counties the board of supervisors appoints as coroner a medical examiner who *is* a physician and a pathologist, usually a forensic pathologist.

When the cause of death is other than natural, only the coroner may sign the death certificate. The coroner must determine who died, when and how death occurred, and by what manner the death occurred—the cause of death. The *cause of death* means a medical disease or condition leading to death. The *manner of death* may be natural causes, accident, suicide, homicide, unknown cause, or equivocal cause. All sudden, unusual, or violent deaths must be reported to the coroner, including deaths which may be natural but where a physician has not recently been in attendance. The coroner's work is a kind of community medicine concerned not only with obviously violent deaths but also with solitary deaths in hotel rooms, crib deaths, and deaths of Jane or John Doe who were too late for the emergency room of the county hospital. The coroner investigates deaths in prisons, institutions, and operating rooms. Accidental deaths of all kinds are coroner cases, however remote the accident is to the time of death.

Laboratory personnel in a coroner's office are often called *dieners. Diener* is a German word that has evolved from its beginning as *a valet* to now as *a servant*, all from the German *dienen* verb meaning to serve. [*Author's note.* When I first heard the term *diener,* I wasn't quite sure what it meant but I quickly adapted to its usage to signify a morgue attendant or morgue assistant. One assistant known as Jess was well educated but from his accent you might not realize he had been a lawyer in The Philippines. One day as we were working on an autopsy, Jess told me that he was curious what the word *diener* meant, so he looked it up in a dictionary. I could not find it in a collegiate dictionary, the *Oxford English Dictionary,* nor in the 1987 English section of unabridged *Random House Dictionary of the English Language Second Edition.* You can, however, in that dictionary find it in the German Dictionary section as valet or servant; and you can find it 1981 *Dorland's Illustrated Medical Dictionary* as a man-of-all-work in a laboratory. A retired physician who worked in the laboratories of University of California San Francisco said he didn't consider *diener* a pejorative term unless you thought that a *diener's* being overruled by his boss was that boss being pejorative. Still, I feel that pathologists might well abolish the use of the word *diener* because it is chauvinistic in its masculinity and current meaning of being a servant. The word *diener* may be ingrained in the vocabulary of the autopsy surgeon, but anyone who can survive the ever-changing terminology of disease can drop the use of the word *diener* for "morgue assistant." To assist at an autopsy may be unpleasant at times but it is not menial. Every morgue worker deserves a title that reflects his status and not his subservience even if the title has more than two syllables. I realize, however, that the word *diener* is still used, and I can't say that forensic pathologists will avoid and discourage the use of the word *diener* in referring to their laboratory personnel.]

Back to what the coroner does: an injury, even if criminally inflicted, does not by itself warrant the involvement of the coroner—the criminally inflicted injury must have caused that death by other than *natural* causes. Also to be remembered is that the coroner does not require a body for investigation, only evidence that a death has occurred.

Coroners are authorized to investigate possible unnatural death without requiring permission of the family. Coroners can take charge of the death scene by locking and sealing the scene. They may direct that an autopsy be performed and may procure body fluids and tissues that they consider necessary to determine the cause and manner of death. If required, coroners may exhume a body or they can amputate and retain hands for fingerprint identification. Coroners can also subpoena witnesses and jurors for the purposes of inquest.

In addition to investigations of unnatural death, California law specifies other functions coroners must perform. They must preserve records of their findings: identification of the deceased; circumstances leading to and surrounding death with names of any witnesses; property collected from the scene and its disposition; persons notified of the death; results of tests both positive and negative; and any opinions rendered by experts in the case. And coroners must inter a body when no other person is available to take charge, but they must not bury indigents in a Potter's Field—a pauper's field—a kind of burial field that would be used only as a free burial ground for strangers, criminals, and people too poor to pay funeral expenses. Also, coroners must perform an autopsy if requested to do so by the family, although the coroner may then charge an appropriate fee.[1]

Coroners' powers are also *limited* by law. They have no jurisdiction in death outside their county, regardless of the county of residence of the deceased. Coroners do not investigate deaths on military reservations or deaths of military personnel in the line of duty. They may retain only those tissues and fluids that are necessary in their opinion to determine the cause of death.

The law specifically permits coroners to retain material necessary or advisable for scientific investigation, but this aspect of the law is not well tested; and most coroners' offices are reluctant to contribute material for research because of possible legal action.

For example, the law permits donation of pituitary glands from coroners' autopsies to the National Pituitary Agency, where the glands can be extracted to produce human-growth hormone for treatment of dwarfism. However, the law also states that the coroner must return the pituitary gland to the body if within 48 hours of the time of the autopsy a subsequently identified relative objects to the use of the pituitary gland for production of the human-growth hormone. Although coroners' autopsies could provide a rich source of human-growth hormone, few offices would care to label separately and *retain* each gland for 48 hours just in case a relative is later identified and the family requests the pituitary returned to the body.[2]

In California, a law now exists that restricts the power of the coroner to retain specimens from cases involving deaths that occur in state hospitals. This law was introduced into the state legislature after a mother complained that the brains of several microcephalic children were, in effect, on display as museum specimens. This law while protecting individual privacy thus could interfere with investigation of deaths in state hospitals. In the long run, this law may thus serve only to obscure from the public the nature of such deaths—and thus a coroner's actions affect the interface of private and public domain.[3]

A coroner's office, however, does not provide an autopsy service simply to satisfy scientific or social curiosity. The coroner's invasion of the property and person of the dead is warranted only as required to protect otherwise unattended persons and to protect the remaining members of society from murder, fraud, and preventable dangers. In order to require an autopsy the law states that in apparent natural deaths the attending physician must be truly unable—not merely reluctant— to sign the death certificate as to cause of death. Still, it seems that some physicians for whatever reason will occasionally attempt to circumvent the desires of the family to avoid autopsy and will report an obviously natural death as unknowable in order to enable an autopsy, perhaps in order to confirm a stated reason that physician has made for the death.

The extent of investigation in a particular death is, of course, determined by the coroner, and it varies considerably among California counties. In a typical community, about 20 to 25 percent of deaths are of a nature requiring notification of the coroner. The coroner, however, may choose to investigate by autopsy only a fraction of cases: coroners may rather consult, at their discretion, a variety of experts, including deputies, autopsy surgeons, toxicologists, criminologists, anthropologists, and dentists.

Funds for coroner investigation are primarily derived from the county, and there are few state resources. Therefore, in cases without violence the coroner may make a death certificate based on relatives' statements and community standards of medical practice. For example, Sudden Infant Death Syndrome (SIDS), also called crib death, is by definition the sudden death of a child less than 1-year-old in which autopsy reveals no cause of death. In such crib deaths the coroner may feel that since autopsy is likely to be unproductive, the case can be expeditiously handled by signing the death certificate without autopsy but in conjunction with a pediatrician. Similarly, a coroner or district attorney for economic reasons may be reluctant to pursue cases in which prosecution is not imminent.

The coroner's inquest is perhaps the most characteristic power of a coroner. Originally an inquest as a legal proceeding was held in the presence of the deceased body. From testimony of witnesses the jurors and the coroner determined the cause and manner of death. The jury and coroner might or might not find criminal and civil responsibility for a death.

Over the years, however, with development in forensic and medical science, and with changes in public attitude, the coroner's inquest became a vestigial remnant of an older system. At the time of this writing in 1980 only a few California counties hold coroners' inquests into deaths.

2

San Francisco Coroners are physicians, beginning 1857.

San Francisco city government originated during the accelerated population growth following the 1849 Gold Rush. "Perhaps never before in the world's history has there been exhibited such a variety and mixture of life-scenes within the same extent and among an equal number of people as in San Francisco for the 2 or 3 years succeeding the discovery of gold."[1]

The situation regarding death in the early 1850s is vividly described in *The Annals of San Francisco* published in 1854.

> Most of the immigrants had arrived in a state of body which was far from sound. The majority came by sea, and had been subjected to all the ills which a voyage of 5 or 6 months' duration usually induces…. There was no record of deaths kept by

authorities, and no examination, inquest, or inquiry whatsoever, was made by them. In the bustle of the place, and continual change of the population, the dead man was not missed…. Friends at the distance of many thousand miles might write dozens of letters, but who could give them information of the missing, unheard of, unseen, unknown emigrant? …. Often the corpse of some unknown was discovered lying in a retired spot, behind some thicker bush than usual, perhaps, or in a remote tent, or at dawn in the public streets. How he had died, whether slain by his own hand or by that of another—whether struck down by sheer hunger, exposure or disease, could often be scarcely ascertained. The man was dead; and that fact was generally enough for the curious.[2]

J M McNulty MD, elected as the fifth Coroner of San Francisco in 1857 was first of the succession of physician-coroners in San Francisco. McNulty later became Health Officer and in 1866 reflected on San Francisco deaths.

We have representatives from almost every clime, with every variety of habits, and were it not for our invigorating climate, the death rate would be largely increased….[3]

San Francisco's municipal government, had been founded mostly by immigrants from northern Europe, and San Francisco government—a city-county setup—included the traditional office of coroner headed by an elected coroner who served a 2-year term. It has been said that life was cheap in pioneer times, but it seems the City did bear the cost of the dead. Collection of the indigent dead, though not to be the only function, was a strong impetus for establishing the San Francisco Coroner's Office.

San Francisco Coroners in the 1850s, however, had more to do than simply collect indigent corpses. In June 1851 the moonlight lynching of John Jenkins in Portsmouth Square became a focus of conflict between City officials and the Citizens' Committee of Vigilance. The case of John Jenkins was the first test of the power of the San Francisco Coroner to hold inquest and thereby determine the cause and manner of death and those responsible.[4]

Following the illegal hanging of Jenkins, which police had attempted to prevent, the body of *alleged* thief John Jenkins was delivered to Mr N Gray, San Francisco's second Coroner and proprietor of a funeral home. Undertaker Gray followed the usual procedure, noting the deceased had $218 in his pockets. Jenkins may have been hanged by someone honest enough to leave money in a dead man's pocket, but the jury impaneled by Gray named nine members of the Vigilance Committee responsible, finding a verdict of death by strangulation.

This decision did not sit well with the Vigilantes, who referred to the "invidious verdict rendered by the Coroner's Jury." The Vigilantes then issued a proclamation indicating that a total of 183 signers were responsible for the hanging, thus consequently obstructing prosecution. City officials were forced for a time to coexist with the Citizens' Committee of Vigilance.[5]

By 1856, 5 years after the Jenkins lynching, the Citizens' Committee of Vigilance, evidently performing its own forensic documentation, publishing a drawing of the entrance and exit gunshot wounds of "Mr James King of William," 34-year-old editor of the *San Francisco Daily Evening Bulletin*. ("While still a youth and because there were several James Kings in his native town [Georgetown, District of Columbia] he assumed [added] the term 'of William,' his father's [first] name, to distinguish himself from the others.")[6]

King had been shot in the left shoulder in the region of the subclavian vessels on the street the evening of 14 May 1856 by San Francisco Supervisor James Casey. One of the first physicians to attend the victim after he was shot was Beverly Cole MD, who developed into one of San Francisco's most colorful physicians. At the age of 23 in Philadelphia, a terrifying pulmonary hemorrhage had destroyed his hopes for the leading medical practice in that eastern city, and he had come to California in search of health—not gold. At the time of the King shooting, Cole was employed as surgeon general to the Committee of Vigilance. (He was himself recovering from an accidental, self-inflicted gunshot wound of the abdomen sustained 2 years earlier in 1854.)[7]

For King's wound Cole *proposed withdrawal of a cloth sponge* that he had at first inserted into the wound to control bleeding (probably because of his wanting to prevent sepsis). The record shows, however, that Cole's care of King for unknown reasons was assumed by "Drs Toland, Hammond, and Bertody," who elected to *leave the sponge in place* for fear of hemorrhage from the possibly damaged subclavian vessels, they said. King died 5 days after the shooting.[8]

Upon King's death, Cole blamed the other physicians of malpractice, claiming that with ordinary care and judgment there would not have been the slightest danger to the life of the wounded man. Although Cole had not been permitted to attend the autopsy he said that the subclavian vessels were not involved in the gunshot wound as described in the autopsy of King performed by Hammond, the physician in attendance when King died. Later, at the inquest held by the Undertaker and Coroner J H Kent who was not a physician, the *San Francisco Daily Evening Bulletin* reported Hammond's autopsy findings.

> ...a ball wound under the clavicle, in the left side, an inch and a half below its middle, passing obliquely upwards to its point of exit on the posterior part of the shoulder blade. I attended Mr King until yesterday, at half-past 1 o'clock, when he died from the effects of the wound. There was no internal bleeding. The principal cause of his death was the violent shock produced at the time of the shot.[9]

Hammond neglected to mention whether the wound involved the pleural space, but one would assume from the location that it had. As attending physician, Hammond was hardly an unbiased observer: one would expect him from his viewpoint to believe that his patient died of the wound and not his treatment. The newspapers mocked the situation.

> Who killed Cock Robin
> I, says Dr "Hammon,"
> With my chloroform and gammon
> I killed Cock Robin
>
> . . . .
>
> Who blabbed the whole?
> I, says Dr Cole,
> It lay on my soul
> And I blabbed the whole.[10]

Casey who shot King was summarily executed 2 days after the death of James King of William. Later,

Police Judge Edward McGowan, implicated in Casey's execution murder, came to trial, permitting a continuance of the battle of the sponge between physicians Hugh Toland and Beverly Cole. At McGowan's trial Cole used a most unusual method of forensic presentation, bringing before the court the somewhat poorly preserved body of a prisoner executed the previous year. Cole used the cadaver to demonstrate the anatomy of the subclavian vessels, a lesson which according to the press the jury did not relish. Cole testified that the wound was not necessarily a mortal one; "and next, the treatment was such as to make it a mortal one." Judge McGowan was found not guilty, that "sponge or not sponge, James King of William had died as a result of a bullet wound inflicted by one James Casey."[11, 12]

In spite of their disagreement over the King case, in 1870 Toland appointed Cole dean of the Toland Medical School, the predecessor to the University of California San Francisco School of Medicine.[13]

Cole was elected city supervisor in 1873 and was instrumental in locating the San Francisco County Hospital (now San Francisco General Hospital) on Potrero Street. In 1895 Cole was president of the American Medical Association, and in 1899 he was elected San Francisco Coroner. He was serving his second term as Coroner when he died of a stroke in 1901.[14]

(Rumor has it that Cole's ashes were originally buried in an earlier Cole Hall at the University of California San Francisco and then later removed to a family plot. However, this story could not be verified.)[15]

3

Some Gold Rush doctors became San Francisco Coroners.

J M McNulty MD, first physician-Coroner in San Francisco, was replaced in 1861 by B A Sheldon MD, a physician for the fire department, who died in office on 19 September 1864. Then San Francisco supervisors chose S R Harris MD from six applicant physicians.[1]

Harris, born in 1802 in Poughkeepsie, New York, trained at New York College of Physicians and Surgeons. Coming to California in 1849 he used a small gold strike to stake himself to a drugstore and medical practice in San Francisco. At that time drugstores had a way of being quite profitable. For example, Dr Hugh H Toland, founder of the medical school now at the University of California San Francisco, made a part his fortune on mail-order diagnoses and patent medicines, sending out aliquots of "anti-syph" and "anti-scrof" remedies by Wells Fargo messengers.[2] But such fortune was not in store for S R Harris MD.

Harris' drugstore and medical office were destroyed by fire. He reestablished his practice after another strike in the gold fields, only to be burned out again. Then, as if ill-prepared for any other livelihood, Harris entered the political arena. A split vote swept Harris into the office of mayor in January 1852 and swept him out again 11 months later. In 1853 he was elected city controller, but after 2 years he returned to medical practice. In 1864 Harris became Coroner and served for 4 years, thereafter returning again to private practice in San Francisco, where he remained until his death on 27 April 1879.[3]

Harris was followed in the office of Coroner by Jonathan Letterman MD. Born in 1824 in Canonsburg, Pennsylvania, Letterman graduated from Jefferson Medical College, Philadelphia. During the Civil War Letterman reorganized the medical branch of the Army of the Republic, serving at many battles, including the Battle of Gettysburg, before becoming San Francisco Coroner in 1868.[4]

Letterman was Coroner of San Francisco during difficult times. During his office, 1868-72, the City suffered a smallpox epidemic. Yellow flags were used to mark quarantined houses, and patients were sent to a smallpox hospital located near Lone Mountain in San Francisco. In 1869 the City spent over $79,000 on smallpox control, and the death toll exceeded the expected number by 100 percent.[5]

The epidemic proved embarrassing for City health officials even though prior to the epidemic the officials *promoted* a municipal vaccination program: failure to vaccinate without medical reason would have been a misdemeanor. Such legal measures had been necessary to enact because the public resisted the smallpox human-source vaccine for fear it might transmit scrofula or syphilis. When the 1860s San Francisco smallpox epidemic struck, the disease had a fulminant onset, not with vesicles—small blisters—but with hemorrhagic purpuric rashes. It seems, at least from the number of admissions to the smallpox hospital, that the 1860s vaccination had done little good. For 968 patients hospitalized with smallpox, 800 gave a history of vaccination by lymph or scab, 40 were not vaccinated, and 128 were of uncertain status. The death rate at the smallpox hospital was 31 percent.[6]

Smallpox deaths did not generally come under the auspices of coroners, but many autopsy procedures were performed in San Francisco at the smallpox hospital. A Dr William H Johnson "made and assisted in making postmortem with the coolness of a philosopher and the anxiety to learn of a student."[7] During the smallpox epidemic, City Health Officer C M Bates complained about the "heterogeneous nomenclature used in reporting the cause of death." Bates cited examples where the cause of death was listed simply as "want of breath," "atropia," or "natural causes."[8]

Deaths from consumption and marasmus—malnutrition occurring in infants and young children—were numerous; and many persons, said Letterman, were too poor to afford a physician or even food. Letterman reported a high rate of death among laborers, and claimed that the "companies who bring these people here should be compelled to take care of them when they are unable to take care of themselves."[9]

Letterman's administration as Coroner is curious in two respects. 1) The low autopsy rate of 7 percent in the first year climbed abruptly to 43 percent in the third year of office.[10] Perhaps during those 2 years Letterman from experience learned the importance of autopsy. 2) Letterman listed *30 accidental* gunshot deaths in 1 year (1869) but later, in 1879, Coroner Levi L Dorr reported *9 accidental* gunshot deaths. Dorr found even 9 accidental gunshot deaths unusually high compared with other major cities.[11] Perhaps Letterman's interpreting so many gunshot deaths as *accidental* showed that during his over-13-years of service as a physician on frontier campaigns against the Seminole, Navaho, and Apache American Indians, he had become calloused to the use of firearms and interpreted all gunshot wounds as *accidental.*[12]

Letterman in 1871 was defeated for the Office of Coroner by J D B Stillman MD. Letterman died in 1872, having been ill for months after breaking his leg in an accident.[13] Stillman's first Coroner's report in 1872 seems to sneer at Letterman's records, calling them "imperfect."[14] Later in 1911, however, Letterman's name was immortalized by the dedication of Letterman Army Hospital in the San Francisco Presidio, presumably more for his military accomplishments than for his successes as a Coroner.[15]

J D B Stillman MD epitomized the Gold Rush character in the Coroner's Office—flamboyant entrepreneur and yet an innovator and academician. Before he came to California during the Gold Rush, Stillman was at one time a staff member at New York's Bellevue Hospital.[16]

In California Stillman demonstrated a flare for forensic medicine even before he came to the Coroner's Office. A crony of wealthy Leland Stanford and Mark Hopkins, Stillman was appointed by Governor Stanford as physician for the then decade-old San Quentin Prison. Stanford's next political appointment of his Lieutenant Governor John Chellis as warden proved embarrassing, but the 1862 debacle gives us a glimpse of Stillman's abilities as a forensic observer.

After lunch on 22 July 1862, Warden Chellis was abducted by 600 convicts from San Quentin Prison, who then escaped with him as hostage to Mt Tamalpais in Marin County across the Bay from San Francisco. Their freedom lasted only until the obese and poorly conditioned Chellis had to be left behind because he couldn't keep up with the escaping prisoners.

Stillman heard of the kidnap-escape while in his San Francisco office. While the fugitives were violently rounded up Stillman hastened to the San Quentin Prison Hospital where he reported on the casualties.

> Brewer was shot through the thigh with a mini-ball which fractured the head of the right femur on its passage out and proved fatal on the ninth week. Bieta, a California Indian, received a shot nearly in the same region. He recovered from his wounds, but died in November of tubercular disease consequent on his injuries. Rodriguez was shot through the lungs with a pistol ball, but is entirely recovered. Blonnel, wounded through the shoulder, had also a buckshot enter the mastoid process of the temporal bone and pass out at the mouth, carrying away portions of the two upper middle incisors. Farrow was shot through the neck from behind, the ball

passing out between the trachea and sterno-mastoid muscle. Both these cases recovered, contrary to my expectations. Twelve [other prisoner cases] were wounded in the lower extremities. One of these, Keller, had his thigh fractured at its middle part by a ball passing entirely through. The chances for saving the man's life were small in any attempt to save his limb, but after mature deliberation upon all the circumstances, he concluded to share the fate of his leg. I respected his determination, and saved his leg, though much shortened.[17]

Stillman was well known for his Gold Rush flamboyancy, but his tenure at San Quentin showed he was also a man of compassion. He spoke out with knowing horror on the treatment of the criminally insane and on the lack of rehabilitative efforts for ex-convicts.[18]

The first San Francisco Coroner to list an autopsy surgeon in his budget, Stillman hired Edwin Bently MD, professor of descriptive and microscopic anatomy at the Medical College of the Pacific (the beginning of Stanford University's School of Medicine). Bently was possibly the first pathologist in San Francisco. Stillman in the early 1870s described the difficulties of antisepsis that plagued these autopsy surgeons. "These postmortems are attended with great danger, and one of my assistants nearly lost his life during an examination" because of a laceration received during an autopsy, with sepsis then setting in.[19]

Stillman's 2-year administration of the San Francisco Coroner's Office was associated with several improvements and legal changes. A new law passed in 1871 clearly stated San Francisco Coroners' responsibilities. 1) Coroners should retain copies of all testimony for inquests and exercise care in selecting jurors for the inquests. 2) Coroners must perform autopsy for homicide cases in front of a second medical witness. 3) Coroners should record and collect personal property and report on its transfer to the City Treasurer, thus relieving the Coroner of some public administrative duties. 4) Provision was made for a $10 reward for bodies recovered from the San Francisco Bay. (Even today "floaters" are a difficult problem for the San Francisco Coroners.)[20]

4

San Francisco faces corruption in the City Morgue.

The first of two major scandals involving the San Francisco Coroner occurred in November 1874 when Coroner John R Rice MD was removed from office by the 12th District Court. Rice had replaced J D B Stillman MD by the 1873 election that had earlier provoked an editorial in *Western Lancet* (forerunner to *California Medicine* and *Western Journal of Medicine*). The editorial criticized Rice, not for his qualifications, but because he was relatively unknown to the community, asking why taxpayers and the Democratic Party insisted on nominating comparative strangers for Coroner. "Why? No one can answer, unless it be, as has been asserted, that a man without any political record will always prove to be a more available candidate and can more easily be elected."[1]

The concerns of *Western Lancet* were well founded.

The proceedings against Coroner Rice, said to be the talk of the town, were further described in the San Francisco *Daily Evening Bulletin*. It seems that on several occasions Rice was casual in summoning jurors. For example, when friends of deceased John Pritchard appealed for permission to remove and bury the body, Rice indicated that as it would be difficult formally to summon a jury in the Western Addition of San Francisco, and the proceedings would be expedited if a group of Pritchard's friends could just be called together for the inquest.[2]

Then, in several cases when the deceased had no relatives, Coroner Rice paid directly for a funeral—with $50 or $60 of the deceased's own money. This was illegal under the law of 30 March 1874, and the *Daily Evening Bulletin* suggested that Rice was receiving compensation from the funeral home.[3]

Finally, there was the case of Dr Amos Farnsworth's robe. When Farnsworth died 26 February 1874, his relatives petitioned the Coroner for a certain distinctive fur robe made up of one California lion skin and sixteen grey fox skins, the coat believed to have been in Farnsworth's possession when he died. Coroner Rice explained that he had an almost identical robe that he had had made up of skins he bought from a street salesman. The robe in question, however, was testified by Mrs Rice as used by her on Christmas Eve. After an elaborate trial Rice was ordered removed from office,[4] a wag might having said that Rice had been removed as a robe-robbing rogue.

A coroner and his deputies can always be subject to temptation for larceny. Scattered throughout the municipal records of the 1870s are examples of rich miners who died with lists of bonds and gold nuggets in their possession. In 1873, based on a law approved 16 March 1872, the City Treasurer received $4092 in unclaimed money, not including other property, and by 1878 the annual amount received from the Coroner's Office was $15,156, an amount even greater than the Coroner's Office total annual budget.[5]

[Even in more recent times, abuses have still occurred. In the 1950s three Coroner's deputies from San Francisco went to prison for criminal activities during investigation of death scenes. A story is told that Coroner Henry Turkel MD suspecting thievery by his own deputies would occasionally plant marked money at a death scene. If the money did not appear on the record, the deputy lost his job. If the money did appear on the record, the Coroner lost his money.[6]]

It was almost inevitable during the early years of the San Francisco Coroner's Office that illicit dealings would develop between Coroners and morticians: until 1881 there *was* no San Francisco City Morgue, and the Coroner was dependent on morticians to provide a facility for autopsy, and sometimes even transportation for the bodies. Coroner Letterman had said back in 1869:

> In a city like this with people from all parts of the world, a great deal of labor devolves upon a coroner—cases involving life depend upon his investigation; and yet he has no office, but must rely upon the courtesy of an undertaker to furnish a morgue, or deadhouse.[7]

Following the 1874 removal of corrupt Coroner Rice, Benjamin R Swan MD was appointed San Francisco Coroner.[8] The new Coroner immediately requested that San Francisco City & County provide a Morgue. In addition, Swan appeared before the 21st session of the state legislature to request a second coroner's deputy. At that time the San Francisco Coroner's Office already had a deputy coroner, an autopsy surgeon, a messenger, and a chemist.

But there was no City Morgue until in 1881 Coroner Marc Levingston MD contracted Undertaker William J Mallady to provide a public "deadhouse" or City Morgue with "all the latest hygienic improvements, such as patent slabs and sprays, asphaltum flooring, and water-tight compartments...." The new City Morgue was located on O'Farrell Street.

In 1884 Coroner Charles Carroll O'Donnell MD reported that the City Morgue had been moved to Washington Street near the Hall of Justice. In the 1884 San Francisco Municipal Reports, O'Donnell notes that the new City Hall then under construction included an area for the Coroner but that the mayor had usurped the space for his own use. When the earthquake struck in 1906 this version of City Hall still was not completed, so we can presume that the earthquake for the time being ended competition for space between the mayor and the Coroner although O'Donnell's reputation for candid behavior later proved unreliable.

After the 1906 earthquake the Coroner's Office was relocated at 363 Fell Street until 1915 when it moved to the second Hall of Justice, the building immortalized by "Ironsides" television program. The City Morgue in the second Hall of Justice was designed by Coroner Thomas B W Leland MD and the City Architect. Since 1961 the Coroner's Office and the City Morgue have been at their present location on Bryant Street in the third and present Hall of Justice.[9, 10, 11]

5

Did William Ralston suicide?

Newspapers, and, particularly, a recounting of the story by George D Lyman MD, a private practitioner of medicine and an esteemed medical historian of San Francisco, relate details around an 1875 impact on forensic science of 19th-century San Francisco: the William Ralston case.[1,2]

Ralston, a wealthy bank and mining magnate—a so-called builder of San Francisco—suffered complete financial loss in 1875. After a board meeting, 27 August 1875, Ralston drowned while swimming in front of the old Neptune Bath House near the present-day Aquatic Park.

After swimming a considerable distance from shore, Ralston had seemed to be in difficulty. Reports varied, some saying Ralston had struggled against the current in the Bay, others saying he went limp. Newspapers reported that Ralston had ingested a vial of poison. A small boat came to Ralston's rescue and brought him ashore. Resuscitation was attempted by chafing of extremities and artificial respiration. Ralston, however, was dead.

The citizens of San Francisco, shocked by the death of such a well-to-do member of the community, turned to Coroner Benjamin R Swan MD for an explanation. Was Ralston's death a result of suicide, accident, or natural cause?

You won't find much in the official Coroner's reports that 1875 year about William Ralston's death in San Francisco's waters. The Coroner's records were destroyed in the 1906 earthquake; but even so, detailed reports about Coroner's-case deaths were not regularly kept until 1928. Before that time you will find in the Coroner's records only a few personal notes kept by the autopsy surgeon for testimony, or short comments penned on the death register page.

Coroner Swan was a well known physician in San Francisco. Once president of the San Francisco Benevolent Medical Society, forerunner to San Francisco Medical Society, Swan also contributed to medicine as librarian and curator of the pathology museum for his society.[3] After removal of corrupt Coroner John Rice MD, physician Benjamin Swan, facing strong competition, sought and gained appointment from the San Francisco Board of Supervisors.

Former Coroners McNulty, Harris, and Stillman had also been on hand, each hoping to regain his old job. And the Tax Payer Coalition had the usual dark horse nomination, a Doctor Grover. The competition was largely between Benjamin Swan MD and Gold Rush J D B Stillman MD. Swan won after his statement "I am not committed to any man, society, clique, or undertaker, and I make no promises concerning appointment of subordinates or Morgue patronage."[4]

Something of Swan's forensic work and that of his autopsy surgeon and chemist are revealed in the following account of the William Ralston inquest from the *San Francisco Daily Evening Bulletin* of 31 August 1875.[5]

> At 1 o'clock this afternoon, the inquest upon the body of William C Ralston was resumed at the Coroner's Office. Coroner Swan stated that the chemist, Louis Falkenau, had not completed the analysis of the contents of the stomach. The process was slow, and he [the chemist] had been laboring night and day....
>
> *Juror* – How long will it take?
>
> *Coroner* – 3 or 4 days.
>
> *Col Barnes* – I suppose you propose to test the stomach for every species of poison?
>
> *Coroner* – There are certain rules for the proceedings of chemists. I think the analysis will be completed by Friday.
>
> *Mr Cohen* – Was the stomach removed by you?
>
> *Coroner* – Yes; by Dr Crook and I [sic]. I sealed it up and gave it to Mr Falkenau.
>
> *Mr Cohen* – Is it the usual custom in cases of this kind, where so much of importance is involved, to submit the stomach to one chemist?
>
> *Coroner* – Yes. I appointed Mr Falkenau for that purpose.

Mr Cohen – I understand from medical juris-
prudence that the examination should be
made in the presence of a witness.

Coroner – In criminal cases perhaps that
should be so, but this is a simple inquiry, to
test the fact of how the deceased came to
his death.

Mr Cohen – I understand that there is a very
large amount of life insurance in this case....
I should think it prudent under the circumstances not to confine the analysis to one
man. It appears to me that no prudent public
official would accept such responsibility....

Mr Weller – Let us have the testimony and be
guided by it....

Dr John T Crook [autopsy surgeon] presented the
following report of the result of the postmortem
examination.

San Francisco, 29 August 1875, [to] Benjamin
R Swan MD.... Herewith please find report of
postmortem examination made this morning
by your order.

William C Ralston aged 49, a native of the
United States, who died 27 August [in the
afternoon].... Autopsy about 17 hours after
death.

External examination: body of stoutly built
muscular man, well developed and nourished;
rigor mortis strongly marked; pupils of both
eyes slightly irregular; face, neck, and upper
part of breasts livid, mottled from postmortem
discoloration; abrasions of the skin of the face,
chest, arms and legs. The abrasions were
recent and of no importance; wet sand
between the toes and under the nails of

both feet; no other signs of injury or violence on external surface of body. Under the scalp, great congestion of the tissues, several auricles of blood escaping on making the sections.

Cranial cavity: dura mater very dense and adhering to calvaria [domelike superior portion of the cranium], and its sinuses engorged with blood. Pia mater slightly injected and covering a small amount of clear serum, most marked at the apex of the right hemisphere, at which point was also a small stain of extravasated blood. No general congestion observed; was most markedly a vaneus [sic] congestion. The external system and substance of the brain itself being rather anenic [sic]. The brain was large in size, fully developed, and its substance firm. No serum in ventricles; abnormal in amount. The cerebellum and medulla normal. The quantity of fluid, blood, and serum, after section of vessels surrounding the brain, I estimate about 4 ounces. No fracture or injury to cranial bones.

Thoracic cavity: Both lungs greatly distended, filling the whole cavity of thorax, thin lower lobes and posterior portions moderately congested; they were crepetant, and with the exception of a slight old adhesion and a small cicatrix at apex of right lung, were healthy and normal. The various membranes of trachea and bronchi were congested and covered with frothy blood-stained mucous. No water was contained in quantity sufficient to be recognized.... Pericardium, heart valves, and vessels normal and healthy; right heart and vessel into it contained fluid blood.

Abdominal cavity: stomach and intestines greatly distended with gas; stomach slightly congested, containing about 1 ounce grumous fluid, its mucous coat slightly injected and softened; small and large intestines normal and healthy, and comparatively empty; liver, spleen, and pancreas normal; both kidneys and portal system moderately congested; bladder contracted; blood fluid throughout the body. Stomach removed for analysis. Immediate cause of death, asphyxia with cerebral congestion.

Col Barnes – Please read the part relating to the stomach over again.

The Coroner read as directed.

Barnes – Now, Doctor, please give in plain language the condition of the body.

Dr Crook – There were no indications of disease except the apex of the upper lobes of the right lung had at a former time adhered to the wall. With that exception there was no appearance of disease. The inability to expel air from the lungs prevented the return of blood. The lungs were full of blood.

Mr Cohen – Then the indications were that death was not caused by drowning?

Dr Crook – Yes, he died from asphyxia. Sometimes a person dies from shock. People die from two causes—from a shock or from asphyxia, as completely as if a string was tied about the neck.

Mr Cohen – Was there any appearance of death having been caused by anything taken into the stomach?

Dr Crook – Nothing that the eye could discover.

Col Barnes – Was there no inflation of the lungs?

Dr Crook – No, none whatever. I opened the stomach, and put it into a jar, which I opened in the chemist's office. There was only about an ounce of fluid in the stomach.

Col Barnes – Were the intestines empty?

Dr Crook – Yes; showing that recently but little food had been taken.

Coroner – Dr Sawyer witnessed the autopsy at my request. Drs Eckel and Haynes were also present a part of the time. At the next inquest I will produce these gentlemen, if you wish to ask them any questions.

Mr Keen – In your opinion, Doctor, could any poison be taken into the stomach and produce the effect upon the brain without leaving a coating on the stomach?

Dr Crook – Yes; some substances. A preparation of opium rarely leaves a mark on the stomach.[6]

Autopsy Surgeon Crook's report is probably the most complete autopsy report from the San Francisco Coroner's Office before 1928, partly of course because of destruction of documents by fire after the 1906 earthquake.

Crook's autopsy was performed in the style of Rudolph Virchow, then contemporary German medico-legal pathologist, who in the same year published his classic *Postmortem Examination with Especial Reference to Medico-Legal Practice.*[7] Virchow emphasized the importance of observing the quantity of blood at various sites, and considered the distention of the right heart to be characteristic of asphyxia.

To this day the manner of Ralston's death is a subject of confusion. Autopsy Surgeon Crook's testimony as written in the *San Francisco Evening Bulletin,* 31 August 1875, is contradictory and somewhat difficult to interpret. He states the cause of death as asphyxia, but appends "with cerebral congestion." Coroner Swan's inquest jury, selected entirely from among the dead Ralston's friends, determined that cerebral congestion was indicative of a stroke.

The New York Life Insurance Company settled with the wife on the basis of a natural death.[8]

6

San Francisco chooses its first forensic scientist.

The origins of forensic science in America are usually traced to the New England area. The first state to require that its coroners be physicians was Massachusetts, passing a law in 1877.[1] By that time San Francisco had already established a *tradition* that its Coroners should be physicians: after 1857 all San Francisco Coroners were MDs.[2]

For 1878, San Francisco elected as Coroner a brilliant practitioner and active forensic scientist, Levi L Dorr MD, establishing San Francisco beginnings of a renown forensic-science tradition. Dorr was born in 1840 and graduated from New York College of Physicians and Surgeons in 1866. He came west after internship at Bellevue Hospital.[3]

The *San Francisco Municipal Reports* began in 1859, and in 1931 were renamed the *San Francisco Municipal Reports Blue Book.* These volumes contain a yearly report by the Coroner—budget analyses, mortality statistics displayed in various ways, and typically a few miscellaneous comments. After 1972, with a tradition started by Coroner Boyd Stephens MD, the Coroner's Annual Report is in a separate volume.

From the *Municipal Reports* one can learn that during the early years San Francisco Coroner's Office handled between 100 and 400 cases each year, with autopsies performed variedly in 7 percent to 50 percent of these cases. The number of cases investigated by the Coroner generally increased in proportion to the population increase. In almost every year accidental deaths outnumbered suicides, and suicides exceeded murders. These proportions were still true in 1978.[4]

During the early years of Coroners' reports, drowning and fire were common causes of death. Deaths due to alcoholism or opiate poisoning have always been common. However, there was over a 7-year period during the late 1800s a remarkably low percentage of deaths due to cancer, cited by the then Health Department as 1.6 percent of all deaths. In contrast, jumping ahead to the *year of 1978, 71 percent of all deaths* were caused by cancer.[5]

Coroner Levi Dorr MD initiated considerable controversy with his solution to relieve the City of some of the financial burden of autopsy. The Coroner's budget allowed $20 per autopsy, and Dorr's office performed nearly 200 autopsy procedures per year. To save the City that $20 per autopsy, Dorr encouraged the law of 1877 that permitted the Coroner to enlist the already paid services of the police surgeon or city physician to perform the necessary postmortem examinations. With the new law, the Coroner could even direct private-practice attending physicians to do an autopsy if they were unable to sign the death certificate as to cause of death.[6]

The Coroner's Office under Dorr kept detailed reports, carefully describing the features of the unknown dead as well as the locations where these bodies were found. And Dorr refused to identify a dead person only on the basis of papers found on the body. From his death records Dorr compiled statistics of suicide, accidental death, murder, and alcoholism; and for wider medical readership these statistics were published in varied medical journals outside the *San Francisco Municipal Reports,* the usual archive for the San Francisco Coroner's records. Dorr was the first San Francisco Coroner to publish his forensic experiences.[7, 8, 9, 10] In these medical journals Dorr described nicotine and potassium-bromide poisoning, rabies, and tracheostomy for extraction of a foreign body.

Homicides in 1880 were more common in San Francisco (1 per 11,190 people per year) as compared to New York (1 per 25,000). A high frequency of suicide has always characterized San Francisco, and in 1880 Dorr found the most common suicide profile to be a single European emigrant male between 20 and 40 years old with no relatives in the State of California. In 687 suicides, 30 percent were committed by gunshot and approximately 15 percent were due each to strychnine, opium, strangulation, and knife wounds. Dorr reported that the introduction of illuminating gas was associated with extraordinary mortality, both by suicide and accident. Unlike natural gas, illuminating gas contains carbon monoxide.[11]

Dorr touted a curious suggestion to prevent suicides, referring to a comment at the International Medical-Legal Congress in Paris. He thought that the only means to diminish suicides is to give their bodies to anatomical amphitheaters.[12] Perhaps Dorr believed that live people would not want to think of their dead bodies being on exhibit, and that thought would serve as a deterrent to suicide.

In response to a perceived challenge that all San Francisco Coroners' cases were due to alcoholism, Dorr performed a prospective analysis of 152 coroner cases. In fact, Dorr wrote in his annual report, only about 1/3 of the 152 cases were directly due to the effects of alcohol, not nearly as high a percentage as one might have expected.[13]

Coroner Dorr was a strong advocate of the autopsy. Speaking in the *San Francisco Municipal Reports* of 1881 Dorr said

> ...the strange or mysterious deaths were about the same, and only to be explained by this desirable custom of examinations after death. By these means [the autopsy] many persons have been relieved of all suspicion from possible crime, and unknown or hereditary diseases have been discovered.... In these days of life insurance and cooperative beneficiary societies, when it becomes necessary to exclude a possibility of fraud, autopsies are more general, and less objected to by friends and relatives. If autopsies were more generally resorted to by the general practitioner, this office would be relieved of some of its work in a matter of the greatest interest to those who have known, examined, and perhaps treated the cases during life.[14]

Western Lancet applauded Coroner Dorr's support for the autopsy, taking an even stronger position.

> We look forward to the time when cremation will have been generally adopted and an autopsy before cremating the body made compulsory.... Then the careful, painstaking physician will be recognized and perhaps some of the lights of the profession might not always shine so brilliantly.[15]

The first year that a Coroner listed an autopsy surgeon in his budget was 1871. For 1878 Coroner Dorr listed three autopsy surgeons. Then there was Dr Blach, German-trained City physician, who served as autopsy surgeon for 11 years. There were also many police surgeons who worked in the Morgue, including George B Sommers MD who later wrote many articles for *California Medicine,* and Thomas B W Leland MD who later became Coroner. The duty of performing medical-legal autopsy examinations for San Francisco fell upon the police surgeon and City physician, and remained there until at least 1900.[16]

Not everyone, however, regarded the autopsy as the proper responsibility for a police surgeon or City physician. Perhaps the controversy explains Dorr's leaving forensic pathology after two terms as Coroner. In 1882, while still in his early 40s, Dorr returned to the private practice of medicine in which he remained until his mid-80s. He died in 1935 at the age of 95.[17]

Subsequent to Coroner Dorr, Coroners F L Weeks MD and Marc Levingston MD bitterly protested the conflicts of interest entailed in doing autopsies.

> A moment's reflection will suffice to show the improprieties of a surgeon who holds postmortem

examination almost daily at the Morgue (some
of the bodies being in an advanced state of
decomposition), of [then] leaving his work and
hastening to the city receiving hospital, and there
proceeding to dress fresh wounds.... The paltry sum
saved by fixing the duties of performing autopsies
for the Coroner on the police surgeon are not worth
considering when such terrible results might follow.[18]

Although the possibility of infection was emphasized, the basic question was whether the police surgeon
should perform an autopsy on a patient he himself had
treated, as when Dr Hammond in 1856 performed an
autopsy on his private patient James King of William—a
case hotly debated in the local press.

In 1882 following Coroner Dorr's years, the forensics attention of Coroner F L Weeks MD focused on his
20-year review of homicide in San Francisco, including
393 cases with 117 cases due to gunshot wounds. Weeks
commented that there "...are so many in our midst
...who do not consider that their toilet is complete for
evening's walk or to call upon a friend unless they have a
revolver hung to their sides."[19]

Weeks then in addition to recommending laws con-
trolling firearms sought more stringent pharmaceutical
laws requiring registration for sale of poisonous drugs.[20]

The next Coroner, Marc Levingston MD, continuing
the forensics interests of Dorr, introduced the practice of
photographing the unknown dead for later identification. In addition Levingston emphasized the importance
of public education in preventing the rising number of
deaths associated with illuminating gas: "...since the
late reduction in the price of gas...people who were
theretofore unaccustomed to its use...and not knowing

the fatal consequences[,] extinguished the gas by blowing it out."[21]   Levingston also reported on the dangerous conditions of some wharves where even horses had fallen through large holes in the planking.[22]

Coroner Dorr and his successors Weeks and Levingston introduced the academic and scientific aspects for forensic medicine: they contributed to the growth of San Francisco as a center for medical study on the West Coast. Although sometimes overshadowed by medical centers in the East, at least some of the origins of forensic medicine in America can thus be traced to San Francisco.

7

San Francisco suffers its worst Coroner.

San Francisco's worst Coroner was Charles C O'Donnell MD. The *San Francisco Chronicle* had alledgedly maligned O'Donnell when he earlier ran for Coroner, publishing an article saying that during the Civil War O'Donnell "often cut off the arms and legs of the wounded prisoners in order that they might not be able to again fight the confederacy."[1]

The *Chronicle* supposedly had noted that O'Donnell had also been found guilty of abortion on numerous occasions. These accusations led to O'Donnell bringing a libel suit against the *Chronicle,* but he reportedly impeached himself during testimony. "I am not a graduate of any medical college. I would not swear that I did not tell people that I had been in the Army of Virginia, and had cut off the legs of Union soldiers to disable them from service." When shown his statement that he was a graduate of Dartmouth Medical College, O'Donnell was stated to have denied it was his own signature on the statement, later admitting he had "written it in fun."[2]

The 1883 election of O'Donnell to the office of San Francisco Coroner was indicative during an era when San Francisco suffered vicious anti-Chinese actions. O'Donnell had campaigned for the Coroner's Office on a platform blaming the "coolie slaves" for flooding the labor market, and crediting them directly for unemployment, poverty, and suicides. O'Donnell, for example, just before his election was arrested for having exhibited to the public gaze a "loathsome object in the shape of a Chinaman suffering with elephantiasis."[3]

The Chinese population had long been subject to blame by health officials. Earlier in 1866, a City Health Officer lamented the Chinese problems.

> Another prolific source of disease is the crowded and filthy condition of our American-Chinese population. So long as they are permitted to occupy the miserable and rickety old shanties in the very heart of the City, this will be an injury to public health, and a shock to decency.[4]

In 1871, Health Officer C M Bates MD *omitted* Chinese-Americans' mortality from San Francisco "statistics," claiming to "demonstrate, by unmistakable facts and figures, that the worldwide notoriety of our healthy and exhilarating climate is fully justified[,]…. …establishing the salubrity of our climate.…" From these doctored statistics Bates thus established that mortality in San Francisco was lower than in any other major city in the United States.[5]

The Chinese-Americans along with their custom of smoking opium were censured for everything from fires said to arise from Chinese laundries to high 1893 violent-death rate of their people in San Francisco, tabulated as 1 per 1200 "Mongolian Nativities" compared to 1 per 19,000 non-Mongolian Nativities.[6] Murder, opium, and the death houses of Chinatown must have been a problem for the Coroner, but it is interesting to note that not until 1892 did the Coroner's budget include a substantial fee for an interpreter.[7]

As Coroner, Charles O'Donnell tried out his own solution to the Chinese-American population problem— so the San Francisco Grand Jury found. In the 18 May 1886 *San Francisco Daily Morning Call,* the Jury alluded to Charles O'Donnell as

> ...the unpopular office-holder..... ... connected by the Jury with the dynamite conspiracy of last year.... ...but the proof of an overt act was not sufficiently established for indictment. The people...have reason to regret that they have placed such a demagogue in office. We believe this City official's course has injured the good name of San Francisco in the East, and retarded this community in getting cooperation and relief on the Chinese question from that quarter.

> The Jury regretted that the statute was not broad enough to allow the filing of presentments for removal from office in such cases and hoped it would be amended to meet them hereafter.[8]

The case of Cecelia Bowers in 1885 added to the disgrace of Coroner Charles O'Donnell.[9] Cecelia Bowers had died after prolonged illness. It was believed that Mrs Bowers was poisoned by her husband, J Milton Bowers MD, suspected by the police to be an abortionist.

Dr Bowers agreed with a deputy coroner that he would not bury his wife until a suitable inquest was held. Nevertheless, the body was buried, Coroner O'Donnell's signature appearing on the burial permission. Strangely, none of the witnesses listed on the certificate could remember signing the document.

Later, a railroad man, J Meredith Davies, testified in court that he had overheard Coroner O'Donnell asking Dr Bowers who should be selected for the jury holding inquest over his wife's death. Davies said that Dr Bowers then produced a list of juror prospects. After this testimony at the trial, the *deputy* coroner had the body of Mrs Bowers exhumed.

The autopsy after exhuming Cecelia Bowers was attended by six physicians, all of whom testified at the trial. Four doctors found no anatomic cause for death, but two testified that natural causes were responsible. A white coating was noted in the mouth and on the mucosal surface of the esophagus, and the gastric contents had a garlic-like odor.

The stomach and its contents were delivered to William Johnston MD, physician-chemist for Cooper Medical School (forerunner to Stanford Medical School). Johnston ran the Mitscherlich test for poisonous phosphorus. The presence of phosphorus was indicated: gastric contents were acidified and distilled in the dark, and the distillate in the receiving flask was luminescent.

Other physicians testified that the white coating in mouth and esophagus was calcium. They claimed that the Mitscherlich test could be falsely positive for poisonous phosphorus if phosphate salts were present. Physician-chemist Johnston had prepared for this possibility: he had analyzed the contents of four stomachs from patients treated with phosphate salts prior to death, and he found the Mitscherlich test for phosphorus negative. Johnston even employed a medical student to ingest and regurgitate phosphate salts to illustrate to the jury the salts' harmlessness.

Also at the trial, Albert Abrams MD, demonstrator of pathology at Cooper Medical School, and author of a large number of articles on pathology, including "Methods of Gastric Analysis," presented the liver and heart from the autopsy of exhumed Cecelia Bowers. By microscopic examination, Abrams demonstrated the presence of fatty change in these organs. Jurors could observe a white precipitate, probably phosphorus, which had formed on the surface of the tissues over several days, and which had a characteristic alliaceous or garlic-like smell.

After these varied medical opinions were rendered in court as to the cause of death of Cecelia Bowers, the jury ignored Coroner O'Donnell's original "opinion" and found J Milton Bowers guilty of murder. He was sentenced to hang. The Bowers case is written up in *San Francisco Murders* as "The Case of the Phosphorescent Bride."[10]

(The Mitscherlich test is still considered valid, but yellow phosphorus is no longer commonly used in rat poisons, matches, or fireworks—partly because of the observations of various coroners over the years.)

Charles O'Donnell's damage to forensic medicine ended in 1886 when the electorate removed him from office after his first term. O'Donnell remained in political life, however, running for offices such as coroner, mayor, and governor, but never again elected. He was still on the ballot for Coroner in 1909.[11]

8

San
Francisco
Coroner turns to
public-health
issues.

By the late 1800s the Coroner's annual caseload approached 1000—about one-half as many as at the writing of this history, 1980. During the first 1900s decade, a measure of forensic science's quality is illustrated by the autopsy rate for unusual, sudden, or unexplained deaths, as having *increased* to 93 percent.[1] And an 1898 Victorian comment reflected the mores of San Francisco: Coroner Edward Hill MD hired Grace Harris as matron to the Morgue, saying it was "a disgrace to this community that a public Morgue, where the dead bodies of women are received, was not, in the interest of decency, supplied with a woman to attend such cases."[2] This statement may have in part been an oblique reference to San Francisco Coroners' duties caused by anti-abortion beliefs: deaths by then-illegal abortions, performed both by physicians and non-physicians, occupied a major portion of the Coroners' time.

Closing out the 1800s as Coroner was the faithful Beverly Cole MD, first appearing in this history as a key physician in the controversial 1856 James King of William assassination. Shortly before his death in January 1901, Cole had one last chance to take a another controversial stand—whether bubonic plague existed in San Francisco. His views were published in the 1900 proceedings of the California Academy of Medicine.

> Dr Beverly Cole: ....anybody who thinks that Chinatown today is filthy ought to have seen it in my time. Then it was worth while taking a visitor there. The best places to show have been closed up. The underground holes that I used to revel in and to which I used to take Eastern visitors are gone. The last time I was in Chinatown, 4 or 5 years ago, I was disappointed at the change, and yet, with all the filth and all the nauseating circumstances surrounding it, there never has been an epidemic in Chinatown at any time. Yet we have had epidemics of smallpox several years ago and not a single case was traced to Chinatown. There you will find bubo and smallpox and all kinds of sporadic cases, but I never saw an epidemic in Chinatown. I believe I could find lepers there today, but as to whether there is an epidemic is another thing. The one way in which I could account for it is that in all my experience at the Morgue there never was a Chinaman brought there who was not perfectly clean in his person. His clothes might be dirty or he might have dirty surroundings, but their religion requires them to take a thorough ablution once a fortnight, which, no doubt, he does more frequently on his own account.

Furthermore, in nine cases out of ten, I never saw a clean white man brought in.[3]

Cole proved to be wrong about the bubonic plague not being in Chinatown: the impressive postmortem evidence, including over 90 marshaled autopsies that proved the existence of bubonic plague, was the work of a Dr Kinjoun and his associates at the United States Marine Hospital, forerunner of the US Public Health Hospital [dismantled shortly after 1980].[4]

The remarkable thing about Cole, someone supposedly said at the time, is that he did not die with his boots off. After 50 years of service to the community, while serving as Coroner, Cole at the age of 72 was felled by a stroke, January 1901.[5]

And, the story goes, on the day that Cole died, a young police surgeon Thomas B W Leland MD had testified in court; and he was appointed Coroner at that time by Mayor J D Phelan. *San Francisco Municipal Records* verify that Leland served off and on as elected Coroner for the next 40 years with 2 absences (1906-08, 1910-12).

Under Leland's direction, the Coroner's Office evolved to a form similar to the 1980 Coroner's Office. From Coroner's Reports through the Leland years, it is evident that Leland took great pride in the function of the Coroner's Office. In 1915, having visited coroners and medical examiners throughout the United States, Leland maintained that San Francisco had a model system.[6]

Leland when he took office was a 30-year-old native Californian, born in Jamestown, Tuolumne County. He had graduated from Cooper Medical School in San Francisco in 1894 and had served as a naval surgeon for several years after his internship. In the tradition of San

Francisco Coroners, Leland was a physician, but his specialty was not pathology, and he maintained a private medical practice outside the Coroner's Office. In 1915 he was appointed professor of internal medicine and assistant chairman of physiology at the University of California San Francisco.

Defeated for Coroner by William J Walsh MD in the 1906 election, Leland was not without plenty to do. Immediately after the 1906 earthquake, Mayor Eugene Schmitz appointed him camp surgeon for the disaster. So, while Leland cared for the living, Walsh cared for the dead.[7]

Using San Francisco Medical Examiner-Coroner's Office *Death Reports,* which began again after the 1906 earthquake, you find a medical account of the 1906 earthquake and fire.[8]

There were no postmortem examinations recorded on the day of the quake, 18 April 1906. On the following morning, pathologist Ostroilo S Kucich MD without autopsy began examining bodies brought to the Morgue. In the first hour he examined 6 subjects. The next 57 cases are listed as being examined at 10 o'clock, and then the books show no more death records until 24 April. Kucich would have had to work quickly indeed on the day of the quake because the Morgue, then located in or near the old Hall of Justice, burned to the ground that afternoon. The Coroner's Office personnel fled with the *Death Reports* for April and the Office's *Book of the Unknown Dead.*

What happened to the bodies that must have accumulated at the City Morgue after the earthquake, but before the fire, is inferred from the sequence of the pages in the *Death Reports.* On 25 April 1906, *Death Reports* state that 24 cases were exhumed from Portsmouth Square, which is near the site of the old Hall of Justice. These 24 cases probably had been delivered to the Morgue, but could not be evacuated before the disastrous fire following the quake and hence had been quickly buried after the fire, almost just across the street.

All told, there are 420 deaths registered by the Coroner as having occurred on 18 April 1906, which of course does not include deaths not registered. Most of these bodies were received before 1 May, but 38 bodies were discovered after this date. Victims continued to be found in the ruins of buildings for up to a year. The time of death was listed as 18 April regardless of when the body was found.

Almost half the 420 persons buried were without identification. Methods of identification were often circumstantial, and sometimes, after digging for weeks among the rubble, relatives might identify a deceased relative because he lay next to his shaving mug. The potential for confusion is illustrated in the following history from a *Death Reports* page, stating that remains found "may be from Girard House which was on the northwest corner of 7th and Howard Streets. Or it may be from the Kingsbury which fell in on the Girard."[9] And 2 children's bones were found 4 months later: "Found...by their father...who identified the remains by finding some of the springs of the lounge that they sleep on near the remains."[10]

For the first 75 cases received after the quake the death register page usually states the cause of death as asphyxia by suffocation or as skull fracture. Most of the later cases state no cause of death. Seven deaths are attributed to gunshot wounds in suspected looters: not until 15 May 1906 did the Coroner consider a gunshot-wound death *unjustifiable* homicide. Looting appears to have been a serious problem: "It seems as though this man was looting and so burdened with plunder that he could not make his way out of the debris and sank exhausted and died."[11]

Regular autopsies were not performed until 1 May. Only about five autopsies were performed between 18 April and 1 May—no doubt in cases of great legal import. Doctors were undoubtedly too busy with the living; and even some alive persons were unattended, as in this sad history: "Died on hill back of City & County Hospital. She was burnt out where she lived. Being sick her husband brought her to City & County Hospital. No room there."[12]

9

San Francisco Coroner finds power in juries.

In 1908 Thomas Leland recouped his position as Coroner, but resigned the office in 1909 to campaign unsuccessfuly as democratic mayoral candidate. Perhaps he felt that mayoral politics were similar to Coroner's Office politics: his platform emphasized civic decency, but he was no real competition to a popular labor candidate.[1]

Leland lost that 1909 mayoral election; but in 1912 he regained the Coroner's Office—by the largest majority in the 6 November 1911 election—where he remained until 1940. (Leland's son Sherman also practiced medicine for many years in San Francisco and was an autopsy surgeon in the 1930s).[2]

Leland's greatest efforts as Coroner were in the area of accident prevention and consumer protection, though this work may have been somewhat politically motivated. Leland took a strong position on many issues and would often direct juries at death inquests to assign responsibility for negligence or attach recommendations for change. There is a collection of such recommendations in a book at the Coroner's Office called *Coroner's Office Statistics.*[3] Each recommendation was stimulated by an unnecessary death, and the scope and number of recommendations is impressive. The Coroner had no power to enforce recommendations or determine guilt, so over the years certain types of deaths drew recurrent comments of a similar nature, such as numerous deaths connected to the unrestricted sale of handguns.

However, Leland's recommendations related to public menaces, and situations could easily be improved: filling old wells, draining ponds, providing safe trains and stations, installing streetlights, and fixing sidewalks. Leland's juries suggested city ordinances for the use of ladders and scaffolds, construction of billboards and flagpoles, installation of skylights and haylofts, and sale of fireworks containing phosphorus. Leland's juries recommended lifeguards at swimming pools, signs about the danger of swimming at Land's End, and first-aid kits at a variety of sites, including ships at sea. The death-inquest juries repeatedly emphasized danger of gas—especially poorly vented heaters, and combined gas-electric fixtures.[4]

These juries asked for more fire alarm boxes and fire escapes, adequate breathing apparatus for firemen, right-of-way laws for fire engines, and establishment of a board of fire prevention. Comments were also made concerning infractions of existing fire-code laws.[5]

After the tragic fire in the St Francis Girls Directory in 1915, in which five persons died, the Coroner's death-inquest jury also charged that the Board of Public Works had previously specified dangerous conditions which were not corrected.[6]

Often the Coroner's juries attached their advice to verdicts concerning accidental deaths among laborers. Over 50 recommendations concerned elevators and elevator shafts, longshoreman practices, electrician protocol; and nearly 100 recommendations concerned railways. There were verdicts commenting on the working conditions of window-washers, trench-diggers, street-cleaners, flagmen, and fumigation workers.[7]

Of course there were the automobile accidents. Prior to 1920 the operation of automobiles was not well regulated: there were no requirements for minimum-driver age, competent eyesight, or even driver licensing. The Coroner's death-inquest juries recommended improved intersections and warnings of various hazards. Between 1912 and 1920 these Coroner's juries asked for over 150 traffic ordinances. And Coroner Leland asked the police to examine vehicles involved in fatal accidents for mechanical defects.[8]

Leland's death-inquest juries also made suggestions to the medical community and Medical Society. Besides the constant vigil over abortionists, these juries deplored hospital doors that could be locked from the inside but not opened from the outside; criticized various surgical misadventures; supported the posting of physician's telephone numbers at public telephones, suggested offering emergency services that were unavailable; proposed surgical operations only after proper consent; and opposed private hospitals' rejection of ill but impoverished sufferers. Death-inquest juries recommended laws requiring anesthesia by qualified persons, laws defining distinctions between dental and general surgery, laws assuring proper labeling of drug containers, and laws mandating registration of sale of poisonous substances. During the rabies epidemic of 1912-13, the death-inquest juries emphasized enforcement of the muzzle law.[9]

Coroner Leland advocated creation of special municipal wards for alcoholics, drug addicts, and insane persons. In 1909 the *San Francisco Municipal Reports* published his view.

> At the present time, alcoholics and those suffering drug habits, such as morphine, opium, cocaine, etc, men who have never committed crime, but with whom the use of alcohol and these drugs is a disease, are compelled by force of circumstances to be taken up by the Police, brought before a Magistrate, and sentenced for periods in the County Jail in order to bring about a possible reform. They are confined in the County Jail for various periods, according to the frequency of offense, and become known as "jailbirds," although, possibly, never having committed a crime.[10]

Deaths in the City jails during Leland's tenure were carefully investigated. Leland wanted the city to employ a physician to determine fitness for incarceration, especially when the arrestee was intoxicated, addicted, or physically injured; and he wanted detained suspects to be searched for potential-suicide instruments.

There were certain deaths which Leland did not aggressively pursue. Of all the verdicts rendered, only one deals with possible police brutality. In that case a police officer shot and killed a suspected car thief who turned out to be an innocent man moving a stalled car. The death-inquest jury returned a verdict that held that while the officer should not be held responsible, in the future the department might detail men of greater experience to such cases.[11] The implication can be made in this case that the inquest was used to exonerate the police officer. Similar inferences of collusion between the police and the Los Angeles Coroner, following the Watts Riots later in 1965, led to profound changes in laws, culminating at that time the many years of agitation for change in California's coroner system.

10

San Francisco rejects change in the Coroner's Office.

In 1916 the property tax in San Francisco seemed too high to the Real Estate Board: in that year the Board recruited the Bureau of Municipal Research of New York to evaluate the San Francisco City & County government and devise means to reduce municipal costs. Among other things, the Bureau of Municipal Research suggested that the San Francisco Coroner's Office be abolished because of unnecessary cost and potential corruption. It should be replaced with a medical examiner and Medical Examiner's Office whose purpose was limited to the scientific determination of the cause of death. The installation of a medical examiner in San Francisco, claimed the New York Bureau of Municipal Research, would reduce San Francisco City & County's cost of caring for the dead by 50 percent.[1]

In 1916 the Coroner's staff of 12 consisted of 1 chief deputy, 3 assistant deputies, 2 stenographers, 2 clerk matrons, 1 City Morgue tender, 1 messenger, 1 autopsy surgeon, and 1 toxicologist affiliated with the University of California San Francisco. A medical examiner on the other hand, said the Bureau, would require only 5 staffers: 1 secretary, 1 stenographer, 1 Morgue tender, and 2 matrons. The New York Bureau then concluded that the 1916 budget of $24,220 could be reduced at least by one-half. [2,3]

The New York consultants apparently considered it inefficient that although the San Francisco Coroner was a physician, he did not perform the autopsies. The San Francisco Coroner physician was not necessarily a forensic specialist or even a pathologist and was usually a physician who devoted only a portion of his time to the Coroner's Office. In fact, until 1976 San Francisco's Coroner was not an American Board of Pathology certified anatomic, clinical, and forensic pathologist. History shows that the San Francisco Coroner's position for many years was widely considered appropriate part-time employment of a practitioner who had a private clinical practice, or was slipping into early retirement.

The New York research group also felt that San Francisco Coroners of the early 1900s wielded unnecessary power with potential for corruption, and that they duplicated functions of the courts, police, and district attorney, particularly with their Coroners' juried inquests. The research group reported a related objection that Coroners' inquests carried the weight of legal proceedings but the Coroners were untrained in law.

Altogether the Coroner's jury furnishes a tempting opportunity and an easy means of impeding the administration of criminal justice and of prejudicing the civil rights of interested parties by the simple process of packing a coroner's jury.[4]

However, the 1916 recommendations of the Bureau of Municipal Research of New York were not adopted, probably because the reduced budget had drawbacks. As late as 1958, Coroner Henry Turkel MD defended his budget with probably the same thinking as that of his predecessors in 1916: "Many jurisdictions having seemingly lower cost may be found to have these services provided by other agencies [such] as police, county hospitals, works department, etc, but no less a public expense even if not showing on the Coroner's budget."[5]

Turkel's 1958 yearly per capita cost of operating the San Francisco Coroner's Office was $0.25 per person, and 20 years later in 1978 was $1 per person. (That 1978 $1 was about the same as a round-trip ticket on the municipal railway.)[6]

Further, Coroner Turkel believed that "allowance should be made for the relative standards of practice as reflected in the number of autopsies performed in relation to the total deaths in the community."[7] The percentage of autopsied deaths was at that time one indicator of the standard of practice in a particular locale, and Turkel believed that "allowance should be made for the relative standards of practice as reflected in the number of autopsies performed in relation to the total deaths in the community."[8]

The San Francisco Coroner's Office was critically evaluated again in 1928 when the National Research

Council reported on coroner systems in America. In 1935, Jessie L Carr MD, distinguished pathologist of University of California San Francisco (and after whom the pathology auditorium in San Francisco General Hospital was named) discussed the faults of the system of San Francisco Coroner's Office.

1) The Coroner's Office was elective.

2) There were no facilities for microscopic or bacteriologic studies although the Morgue was **modern and adequate for gross pathology.**

3) **There was no file kep**t for scientific reference.

4) The Coroner was forced to employ an outside histopathologist whose work was accepted only if it pleased the Coroner.

5) No use was made of the vast amount of teaching material available.

6) The cooperation between the Coroner and the legal and prosecuting staff of the City was poor, and cases were frequently neglected because of the trouble necessary in collecting facts for their prosecution.[9]

In pro- and con- *editorials* in that same 1935 issue of *California and Western Medicine,* Carr, pathologist to Coroner Leland, and Oscar Schultz MD, chairman of the Committee on Medicolegal Problems of the Institute of Medicine of Chicago, individually discussed the issue of a coroner system versus a medical-examiner system.

Schultz cited the disruptive effect of a coroner's election on the pursuit of forensic medicine as a career.

> The reason for the failure of the coroner's system to develop a corps of experts is obvious. An elective office with its frequent upheavals and turnovers, and its insecure tenure of office, does not attract

well-trained young physicians into what should be
an attractive and important subdivision of medical
science....The investigation should be of the dead
body for the purpose of determining in as accurate
and as scientific a manner as possible the cause of
death.... All other investigations which have to do
with the detection, apprehension, and punishment
of those who may have a criminal or negligent
responsibility for death should be left to police
agencies, the grand jury, the prosecutor and the
courts.[10]

Carr in his 1935 editorial explained that since the
1928 National Research Council's report many improvements had been made in the San Francisco Coroner's
Office. Under a grant from the City & County government a laboratory had been established for gross photography, microscopic pathology, and bacteriology. For the
first time gross and microscopic autopsy reports were
typed and bound. An agreement between the University
of California San Francisco and the San Francisco
Coroner's Office permitted exchange of academic support and material. Pathologic specimens were presented
at clinico-pathologic conferences at French Hospital, Mt
Zion Hospital, and San Francisco County Hospital. The
Coroner's Office, largely through the efforts of pathology
professors Henry D Moon MD and Robert Wright MD,
contributed many pathologic specimens to the museum
at the University of California San Francisco.

And in addition, in 1932 a profound change in the
selection of the San Francisco Coroner had then taken
place: the Coroner's Office had been removed from popular election and had become an official Civil Service

appointment subject to the approval of the City-County supervisors.[11]

In 1980 at the time of the writing of this history not all these changes have survived. By 1980 there was little back-and-forth of materials or academic support between the San Francisco Coroner's Office and the University of California San Francisco; and clinicopathologic conferences—pertaining both to the symptoms of disease and its pathology—were no longer presented by the Coroner's Office at San Francisco hospitals. The pathology museum at the University of California San Francisco was defunct. Since the death of Dr Henry Moon in 1976, the affiliation between the San Francisco Medical Examiner-Coroner's Office and the University of California San Francisco had become almost non-existent.

11

San Francisco Coroner increases scope of the office.[1]

Henry W Turkel MD in 1951 was elected Coroner of San Francisco after his myocardial infarction—leaving a busy ophthalmology practice. Though it seemed that he entered the Coroner's Office in retirement, Turkel proved a most dedicated Coroner, serving for 20 years. In nationally published articles Turkel wrote elegant and scientific defenses of the coroner system and the autopsy.[2] And in the tradition of San Francisco, Turkel was a major advocate of death-scene investigation, autopsy, and inquest.

Even though he was a physician, Turkel was not a medical examiner nor a trained pathologist. While Turkel supervised the functioning of the office it was trained pathologist Henry D Moon MD, who was the medical examiner to determine the causes of death. Turkel thought that a medical examiner did not necessarily have a superior commitment to accompanying scientific determination of causes of death. He believed that a medical examiner's personal responsibility for *all* aspects of examination might include some interests that limit the necessary scientific or public-health perspectives; and he therefore preferred what he believed to be a wider-scoped coroner system.

Advocating more objective investigations of the causes of death, Turkel published statistics that coroner systems in California performed more autopsies than medical-examiner systems in the eastern United States. In Turkel's 1950s statistics, 10 California county-coroner systems autopsied an average of 74 percent of the medical-legal deaths, which was nearly *20 percent* of the *overall* community deaths. Five eastern-state medical-examiner systems in contrast autopsied an average of 21 percent of the medical-legal deaths, only *3.6 percent* of the *overall* community deaths.

Coroner Turkel found that coroners' offices were often more thorough in investigating deaths than were medical-examiner systems. For example, by Turkel statistics, postmortem laboratory tests totaled 48 percent of cases in California's coroner system, but totaled only 27 percent in New York's medical-examiner system. One result of this increased testing by coroners was a greater appreciation of the problem of barbiturate abuse. The number of deaths attributed to barbiturate toxicity increased as the percentage of cases analyzed for barbiturates increased, thus giving a more accurate picture of the incidence of barbiturate toxicity.

Turkel also used statistics to show that without autopsy the diagnosis in medical-legal death cannot be accurately established. He analyzed 121 cases in which patients before death occurred were only briefly in the hospital with physicians in attendance only a short time: 45 percent of the attending physicians' clinical diagnoses of the cause of death were incorrect as later determined *after* autopsy. Furthermore, the diagnosis of cause of death listed in non-autopsied cases did not involve the correct organ system in 29 percent of the cases. Similar statistics might exist today for patients who die abruptly after admission to a hospital, but such errors in clinical diagnosis as to cause of death compared to autopsy diagnosis are not a reflection on the skill of clinical diagnosis so much as a reflection on the difficulties in diagnosing the cause of death without the extended investigation of autopsy.

In addition to establishing the value of the larger view of a coroner system, Turkel defended the use of the coroner's deputy to investigate the death scene. The coroner's use of a deputy is a characteristic feature of the coroner system in California. Turkel pointed out that police or physicians are not necessary in the initial phases of investigation of medical-legal deaths. In these investigations physicians are not even necessarily superior to a deputy who is specially trained and who devotes full time to examination of circumstances surrounding death. Turkel said

> ...to be frank and practical, the physician must be very rare who, as a required part of the "at the scene" investigation, would routinely slip his hands into the urine-stained and feces-stained clothing of dead persons in search of identification, personal effects, notes, or other evidence. He must be rarer still who would with regularity make a detailed and

exacting search of the body and the premises in which was found a reeking, vermin-infested corpse, which may or may not be liquefying. These actually are not uncommon findings. In the eyes of most physicians, whether autopsy surgeons or not, these cases are unpleasant enough at the autopsy table, and they are not eager to go to the place of death to examine and inspect before a preliminary preparation of the body has been made....

On the other hand, there is an adequate number of lay investigators whose need and pride in the position is sufficient enough to enable them to tolerate the more unpleasant aspects, however distasteful. Such thorough and painstaking investigation as described is essential, even under the most trying circumstances, if all the information available at the scene is to be found.[3]

A trained lay investigator is especially appropriate for rural areas. Most medical-examiner systems are urban based, and there are not sufficient physicians willing or able to serve as medical examiners in rural areas. For example, Turkel quoted the autopsy rate in medical-legal cases in 1953 as 37 percent for Baltimore and 18 percent in the remaining State of Maryland. Turkel was of the opinion that

...in an area as large as California, for example, it is only with some difficulty that physicians are found who will travel over large counties to do the required autopsies, let alone go beforehand to the scene of every death occurring by violence or injury or under doubtful circumstances. Furthermore, if physicians go to the scene of death to view the body and then order an autopsy, they must wait for the body to be moved to some convenient place and then travel to that place, again over great distances, to perform the autopsy. It can be said, and the statistics support, that this [to-and-fro travel] tends to markedly increase the number of cases signed out on the basis of history and circumstances without benefit of autopsy. This [lack of forensics] is not conducive to impartial scientific investigation into the causes of death.[4]

By 1969 Coroner Henry Turkel was not a well man. He had had several heart attacks before coming to office, but he had done well for almost 20 years. Then things seemed to pile up: he was divorcing his wife, and he lived on his boat—like television's character, medical examiner Quincy—or even in his office. Next, he developed gangrene in his legs. Even after his legs were amputated Turkel came to the office but he couldn't keep up with the work.

But by Turkel's time, 1951, because of the potential for personal and political abuses, the San Francisco Coroner system had an advantage over many other coroner systems: the San Francisco Coroner by long tradition since 1857 was a physician; and now Turkel had been the first Coroner to be appointed under Civil Service, those branches of public service concerned with governmental administrative functions outside the armed services. The San Francisco Coroner was *no longer elected to the Office.*

12

Coroners' inquests are abused.

Whether the coroner was a physician or not, one unique feature characterized the earlier coroner systems: the coroner had the power to hold inquest. San Francisco Coroners, like Thomas Leland MD in the early 1900s, accomplished much good by appropriate use of the inquest. Removing the selection of the San Francisco Coroner from the election process and making the office available by Civil Service examination had advantages, but it also made the Coroner less responsive to the public. In Los Angeles, during the aftermath of the 1965 Watts Riot, the public was angered by the Coroner's abuse of the inquest, leading to major changes in California's coroner system, and particularly in the powers of an inquest.

During that 1965 Los Angeles Watts Riot 32 persons were killed. At the direction of the district attorney, the Los Angeles Coroner held inquest into these violent deaths. Neither the families of the deceased nor their attorneys were permitted to participate in the inquest proceedings, except by submitting material questions to the district attorney who at his own discretion could place the question before the witness.

A typical verdict by the Los Angeles Coroner's jury in 1965 read that the deceased "died of gunshot wounds in the chest, while under the influence of alcohol, and was shot by known police officers while committing a felony...justifiable homicide in the lawful performance of a police officer's duties."[1] Inquest verdicts of this nature had been rendered before, but the *exclusion of the family,* the number of deaths involved, and the implied political motivation were unprecedented. Inquests are intended to determine, for the benefit of the community and the family of the deceased, whether any wrongdoing occurred in an individual's death. After the Watts Riot, more than one inquest verdict reported that the deceased individual himself had committed a crime; and in the verdict a series of allegations and previously determined facts were paraded before the public without opportunity for representatives of the accused to provide defense. The Los Angeles Coroner's verdict in the Watts Riot deaths seemed to be a policy initiated by the district attorney that implied public exoneration and justification of police action.

The Los Angeles Coroner's actions in the Watts Riot deaths focused public attention upon a function of coroners that was judicially weak. The coroner and his jury at the inquest were meant to act as checks and balances for law-enforcement agencies: but because the coroner-jury verdict was only advisory (even though findings at the inquest might hurt an individual's reputation), the coroner's inquest provided no real legal check of other agencies. It is true, though, that the powers of a coroner's inquest in some respects exceeded those of a grand jury: a coroner's jury could make a non-binding accusation that the defendant could not at that time answer in any authoritative form. A grand jury on the other hand allowed defendants a reply. Furthermore, coroners for the most part had no long history of interest in investigating possible police homicides.

Arguments against the coroner's inquest were summarized by James N Adler in the 1967 *University of California Los Angeles Law Review.*

> The coroner's jury being ill-equipped to determine the medical cause of death adds nothing to the information secured by the autopsy. Furthermore, the inquest rarely elicits any new non-medical information. It was designed for an era in which an adequate investigation could be performed by summoning all the residents of the area where the death occurred into one place and asking questions. Clearly, this is no longer practical or even possible in most cases. Elaborate field work which the coroner cannot perform is necessary. In fact, it is common to postpone an inquest until [after] the police investigation is completed....[2]

> ...the inquest is limited significantly in function to conveying the information which has been already collected and analyzed by others. This limitation is a result of latent presentation in the dramatic setting of the court like proceeding.[3]

James Adler's analysis of the coroner's inquest was unfair on several counts. 1) The coroner's jury is no less qualified than any other jury to determine the cause of

death.   2) If the jury fails to understand the medical findings, this is a fault in the presentation of evidence that
can occur in any court. 3) Adler, in his 1967 opinion, discussed at length the officer to the King of England in the
12th Century, whence the name coroner, but Adler did
little to consider the history of coroners in America.
4) Adler also disclaimed the value of the coroner's field
investigations at the death scene. 5) He did not acknow-
ledge that the powers of inquest were already limited by
the California laws of 1955 that prevented a coroner's
jury from naming an individual responsible or from issu-
ing a warrant.

If one accepts Adler's views, the coroners can be
faulted by some because they are not physicians and by
others because they are not judges.

After the 1965 Watts Riot a satisfactory alternative to
the inquest was not discussed. If the Los Angeles
Coroner's system had failed properly to evaluate and
deliberate possible police homicide, the usually suggested
alternative of transferring authority from coroner to the
district attorney or to the police would hardly have
improved investigation.

The critical fault of the Los Angeles Coroner after
the Watts Riot deaths was to exclude the family from participation in the inquest. After all, there are cases in which
the cause of death is unknown or the mode is equivocal.
Who should pass judgment on these cases? Should a single person, medically qualified or otherwise, decide what
significance these deaths have to society?

Interrogation of witnesses by a family attorney had
not been permitted in Los Angeles inquests since before
1926.[4] The Los Angeles Coroner had apparently come to

see himself more as an instrument of law enforcement than as belonging to an institution of social justice.

The coroner's inquest, however, is recognition that the medical history is vital to accurate diagnoses. Medical history is always incomplete, and often, autopsy surgeons work with minimal knowledge of the facts of the cases. The significance of almost any anatomic finding can be modified in the presence of certain historical events. It is not archaic nor impractical to assemble all witnesses or family members who might contribute historic information. It is odd that more medical examiners do not recognize the validity of the inquest and its analogy to standard medical history. Granted that the time of bereavement is not an optimal time, it is sometimes a necessary time to interview the family. Excluding the family from the inquest is unreasonable.

A related issue is whether the coroner should direct autopsy to be performed in cases in which the family opposes examination. The coroner or medical examiner usually has the authority to order autopsy, and this authority has been upheld by the courts. In Birmingham, Alabama, however, the coroner's insistence on autopsy in the single-vehicle accidental death of the daughter of a state legislator caused sufficient anger and resentment that the medical-examiner system was abolished to be replaced by a coroner who could perform autopsy only at the direction of the district attorney. Forensic workers must do what is proper within their legal framework, but they must not lose sensitivity to the interests or possible contributions of the family.

Eventually public anger over the 1965 Los Angeles Coroner's verdicts led the California state legislature in

1969 to enact laws reducing the powers of the coroner's jury inquest.[5] Most counties in California do not at present hold coroner's jury inquests for fear of legal entanglement. The law permits the coroner's inquest jury to find verdicts limited only to death by natural cause, accident, suicide, homicide, equivocal mode, or unknown cause. No description, such as "justifiable," can be attached to the verdict, although recommendations for alleviation of the circumstances that led to the death can be appended. Only in San Francisco, Los Angeles, and a few other counties are inquests regularly held.

At the time of this writing, 6 California counties (10 percent) have a physician as coroner; 33 counties (58 percent) have a sheriff as coroner; and 18 counties (32 percent) have another lay person as coroner. Many California coroners depend upon morticians to provide facilities for autopsy.

Whether California counties should convert to medical-examiner systems is not a serious consideration as of the date of this writing in the early 1980s: there are barely enough certified forensic pathologists to serve these 57 coroners, let alone to serve as medical examiners. The real future problem for California coroners is the availability of local funding. State public-health laboratories are available to coroners but qualified personnel and supplies for investigative field work are not always present.

Therefore, a murder that occurs in a rural area may be analyzed differently from one analyzed in a medical examiner-coroner office. In the end the characterization of an office as medical examiner or as coroner is not as important as the authority, scope, and quality of investigation of medical-legal deaths.

13

Academe flourishes in San Francisco Coroner's Office.

Jesse L Carr MD is the father of pathology in San Francisco as well as a nationally recognized pioneer of American pathology. Carr was not the first pathologist in San Francisco, but he was the first of a new and since-vanishing breed of pathologist who masters all aspects of pathology—including the anatomic, clinical, and forensic work. His energies seemed endless. He was also one of the first pathologists to capitalize on the economic possibilities of clinical pathology. Carr is perhaps the most famous and best loved of the physicians who were involved with the San Francisco Coroner's work. His many students have formally recognized Carr's contribution by dedicating the pathology auditorium at San Francisco General Hospital in his name.[1]

Born of Canadian parents in North Dakota in 1901, Carr's family moved to Porterville, California around 1906. Carr's first great interest was cattle ranching, and his family was one of the first in the Marysville area to strike water by drilling. While in college at the University of California Davis, Carr's interest in veterinary medicine convinced him to try his luck with humans. After Harvard Medical School he interned at New York City Hospital, and then he became a surgical resident at the University of California San Francisco.

Pathology in San Francisco was never the same after Jesse Carr MD. While still a resident in pathology in 1929 he began to moonlight as autopsy surgeon under Coroner Thomas Leland, and he also opened a private clinical laboratory in the surgical office of Wallace I Terry MD on Post Street. During the 1930s depression, Coroner Leland would come to the City Morgue in the morning and find that Carr had already done all the autopsies for the day. Then Carr would rush off to Terry's office where he supervised the morning phlebotomies and cardiograms. Terry appeared for his own office hours in the afternoon.

To open his first laboratory Carr invested $600 for a microscope and photometer, and he made a cardiograph from old parts he found in the basement of the county hospital. Carr also claimed that sometimes on a nice Sunday afternoon he would borrow some block and tackle from the orthopedic department at the University of California San Francisco—and maybe a little fungicide from the pharmacy for dry rot—to use on his sailboat. He always had the equipment back in place on Monday morning.[2]

Jesse Carr MD entered the UCSF department of pathology as assistant professor in 1930. He became chief of pathology at San Francisco General Hospital in 1932, a position he held for 35 years. Additionally, as chief pathologist to the Coroner (1940-47) and later as chairman of the department of legal medicine at UCSF (1947-67), Carr made great contributions to forensic medicine. He published articles on forensic matters such as cerebral hemorrhage in boxers, sodium-fluoride poisoning, experimental postmortem-skull fractures, and sudden death.

Carr's most embarrassing paper, although only in retrospect, is probably "Status Thymico-Lympaticus," published in 1945, a definitive work at that time on the enlarged thymus as a cause of sudden-infant death syndrome (SIDS), a thesis once popular but now rejected.[3]

Carr was the first to recognize death by air embolism introduced by blowing air into the vagina during cunnilingus, an event which seems to lodge in the memory of every coroner's deputy as the "most unique" contribution of the San Francisco Coroner's Office.

In 1944 a young man was arrested and faced life in prison under laws prohibiting oral sex. According to the young man's confession he and his girl friend were drunk and amorous, and decided "to go down on each other.... I drew a deep breath and blew inside her.... When I did this, her arms dropped and she went limp." Carr demonstrated that the cause of death was pulmonary embolism, arising from thrombi in the uterus that contained an early conception. The cervix was slightly dilated. Carr reasoned that the death was due to the entrance of air into the vagina during oral sex. In 1935 Carr and a colleague[4] had described embolism following injection of oil into the urinary bladder, and they must have been struck by the similarity of the findings in the death of this young woman. In court, Carr could have summarily dismissed the findings as those of attempted abortion, but instead he explained to the court that the death was accidental. Eventually, the young man was released. "The man responsible for the act faced the criminal charge of murder, but science and wisdom proved stronger than legal technicalities," wrote Harry Benjamin MD, describing the case in the *Journal of Clinical Psychopathology*.[5]

Thus we find Carr in 1944 taking a modern role for the forensic pathologist, that of explaining deaths that might otherwise seem bizarre and subject to misinterpretation. Blowing air into genitalia during oral sex is dangerous but fairly common, and like autoerotic-sexual asphyxia, is likely to be misunderstood by those who have not heard of such practices. We see that Carr clearly acted as an independent agent rather than as a representative of law enforcement, and he based his interpretation on experience and founded expertise.

Carr was a champion of education both in pathology *and* legal medicine. A devoted teacher who wanted medical students to learn forensic pathology, Carr trained many of today's practicing pathologists at the same time that he managed several clinical laboratories in San Francisco.

In the mid-1950s Carr went to Indonesia where he helped establish that country's first pathology laboratory at the medical school in Djakarta. After the tragic death of his first wife, Carr escaped for awhile to an island in Fiji, but soon he was back in San Francisco.

For San Francisco General Hospital Carr promoted the idea of a pathology building to the San Francisco Board of Supervisors. In the mid-1960s the autopsy service at San Francisco General Hospital had four times the number of cases as at the time of this writing. Carr's plan for the new hospital Morgue was "three tables, no waiting." After his retirement in 1967 Carr hardly slowed down. The octogenarian, sometimes seen at San Francisco General Hospital, talked to personnel or poked his head in the Morgue to see what the latest case was about. He truly was the father of pathology in San Francisco.

Another pathologist of historic interest at UCSF, Henry D Moon MD, claimed to be the first Korean child born in San Francisco.[6] His father, Yang Mock Moon, was a Korean scholar who came to San Francisco in 1903 as a political refugee. Finding no work for a Korean scholar in California, Moon's father was employed as a waiter, farm laborer, ginseng-root salesman, and language teacher. Henry's mother was a Korean picture bride who came in 1913, and Henry was born the next year. If father Moon was a frustrated scholar then he would have to have been pleased by his son's progress. Young Moon was definitely a scholar, and very much the Californian scholar. All told, he spent 43 years in the University of California system.

Henry Moon graduated from San Francisco's Galileo High School in 1932 and went to the University of California Berkeley. Moon's Berkeley graduate work in the department of anatomy, creating a bioassay for adrenocorticotropic hormone (ACTH), set the stage for his lifelong interest in hormones of the anterior pituitary gland. Moon co-authored nearly 100 articles, mostly concerning endocrinology, and he introduced many students to this field of research.

Henry Moon received his medical degree from the University of California San Francisco in 1940, completing his pathology training in 1944. During the war years 1942-44, Moon served as autopsy surgeon to San Francisco Coroner Henry Turkel under his friend and associate Jesse Carr MD who was chief pathologist to the Coroner. During 1944-47 Moon served in the military, and on his return he replaced Carr as chief pathologist to the Coroner. Carr's son Lawrence Carr MD commented that from the time Moon was a medical student he was the heir apparent to Jesse Carr MD.

Henry Moon MD became chairman of the department of pathology at the UCSF in 1956; and he attracted a small but renown group of pathologists to this faculty. Moon was president of innumerable professional societies and twice-visiting professor as a specialist for the United States, first to Korea and then to the Soviet Union. Many pathologists practicing today were greatly influenced by and admiring of Moon.

Moon died in 1976 of nasopharyngeal carcinoma after a prolonged illness. Under Moon the UCSF department of pathology included clinical, anatomic, and forensic aspects. But there began rumblings of greater specialization. The department of medicine, for example, clamored for better laboratory service. And at the San Francisco Medical Examiner-Coroner's Office, Coroner Boyd Stephens MD had himself recently become certified as a forensic pathologist. No longer were there pathologists like Carr and Moon who practiced in all pathology fields.

14

San Francisco Coroner's Office changes its academic relationship.[1]

Until 1971, pathology at the San Francisco Coroner's Office was synonymous with the University of California San Francisco department of pathology. Many people actually believed that Henry Moon MD and Jesse Carr MD were Coroners, rather than pathologists to the Coroner.

Moon as chairman of the department of pathology at UCSF (1956-74) worked closely with his business partner Carr who was chief of pathology at San Francisco General Hospital (1932-67). As pathologist to the Coroner, Moon made careful autopsy studies of the vessels in young adults and children, and reported in the literature a landmark study showing that atherosclerosis can begin at an early age.

One of the Coroner's lab technicians reminisced that Moon ran the Coroner's laboratory with an iron hand and did all the microscopy himself. If the autopsy surgeon sent Moon a section of an obvious pathologic condition Moon would chide the surgeon for wasting everyone's time. On the other hand, Moon seemingly inevitably learned when an autopsy had been made on a disease of particular interest or rarity; and if microscopic sections had not been previously made, then Moon was likewise angry. The technician said that the autopsy surgeon lived in fear of making the wrong choice between sections or no sections.

Another of Moon's coworkers said that Moon hated to close a case if the cause of death was unknown, as though this lack of knowledge was an admission that the pathologist had failed. For example, the diagnosis of sudden infant death syndrome (SIDS) did not sit well with Moon. Sometimes he extensively examined a large number of microscopic sections, finally declaring that he had discovered a small focus of inflammation in the lung, a fibrin thrombus, or some other small sign that the death was natural, thus seemingly exonerating the careful work of a pathologist.

Myocarditis played a part in another example of stories about Moon. Robert Wright MD, professor of pathology, UCSF (1956-76), told the story. Working as a pathology resident in the Coroner's Office, Wright had noticed that several coroner-death cases were diagnosed as due to myocarditis. Wright then collected and further studied these cases, and he presented his findings at a University conference of pathologists. As Wright spelled out his detailed myocarditis findings, he noticed

Chairman Moon sitting red-faced in the front row staring hard at him. Wright felt the audience grow restless. He decided that his detailing myocarditis diagnoses was reflected as criticism of Moon's more general myocarditis diagnoses. To make matters worse, next, an older pathologist not realizing that the original general diagnoses had all been made by Moon, unwittingly embarrassed his chief by complaining that merely finding a minute focus of scant inflammatory cells in the myocardium did not necessarily prove a cause of myocarditis death. Then Wright felt that everyone in the audience was embarrassed for Chairman Moon. Wright claimed that he felt that Moon would never again speak to him, but certainly Wright's career under Moon at the University did not seem to suffer.

Another story told by a staffer that illustrates the tenor and interests of getting all the facts in the then Coroner's Office: Robert Wright MD once, when brought the mangled body of an old man run over by a trolley car, realized that the old man had also been beaten. Sure enough, later after investigations, witnesses reported that some thugs had thrown the old man under the trolley after beating and robbing him.

And on another case, Professor of Pathology Robert Wright was chosen to perform the controversial second autopsy on prisoner George Jackson who died at San Quentin Prison and whose cause of death was controversial.

Pathologist Wright even served as a bit actor in the movies—he can be seen dictating an autopsy in the actual San Francisco City Morgue in the 1968 movie *Bullitt* that starred Steve McQueen.

There was a period when movies several times used the actual City Morgue to lend authenticity, and one technician recalled that after he had suggested that a coroner case would not be lying there on a slab with an immaculate coiffure, the movie director mussed the hair-do and gave a $50 tip to the technician for his idea.

Another Coroner's lab technician said that Wright's most unfortunate case was the one where he signed the cause of death as spontaneous peritonitis, cause unknown. The family was unhappy with the diagnosis and called for a second autopsy report. There the pathologist opened the bowel and found a perforation due to a toothpick. After that, the lab technician reported, you couldn't mention toothpicks to Professor Wright without making him mad.

But there came a change in the close relationship between San Francisco Coroner's Office and UCSF. Helping Coroner Henry Turkel MD were his pathologists Jesse Carr MD and Henry Moon MD who ran the Coroner's pathology section using selected faculty members and residents from UCSF.

A public official in the Coroner's Office some years later wrote the following account which is corroborated by several sources at UCSF and in the San Francisco Medical Examiner-Coroner's Office.

> Dr Turkel, a diabetic, was appointed Coroner of San Francisco. The position was brought under Civil Service with lifetime tenure, affording the holder much job security. Towards the end of his career when the inevitable consequences of diabetes were becoming manifest, he managed to receive disability retirement. Dr Turkel apparently intended to continue running the office while retired, and no qualified

replacement was sought. However, since the position could not be left open indefinitely, Dr Boyd Stephens—a second-year resident in pathology at the University of California—was appointed Coroner. He enjoyed the title and salary of Coroner while continuing to function as a full-time resident in pathology at UC. Dr Turkel subsequently died as a result of diabetic complications, and Dr Stephens remained as Coroner for 2 years, all the while in full-time training at UC. Thus, the position of Coroner was considered by some to be a highly paid moonlighting job for a resident in pathology.

In order to avoid being drafted into the military while in training, Dr Stephens joined the Barry Plan—a voluntary commitment to the Navy. [An enrollee would make a voluntary commitment to the US Navy and not be drafted into the military while in training.] When he [Stephens] neared the completion of his residency at UC, and his service obligation was imminent, he turned to the Board of Supervisors of San Francisco to get his service deferred on the basis that his absence (from his avocation as Coroner) would work a hardship on the City & County of San Francisco.

The San Francisco Board of Supervisors chose not to recognize Stephens' draft into military service as a hardship to San Francisco; and if Stephens entered the military from the position of *acting* Coroner he would not necessarily be able to return to that office. However, if Stephens were to be appointed *full* Coroner before he went into service, then under selective service regulations Stephens' deferment would be extended until he completed a probationary period in that office as full Coroner.

Records show that in 1972 a Civil Service examination was held for the San Francisco Coroner after a small newspaper announcement—a typical procedure for any Civil Service position. At that time it was not traditional to make an attempt to recruit pathologists outside California, as it would by law be today. The Civil Service newspaper announcement stated that the examination would be given when "the number of qualified applicants warrants the holding of a competitive examination." Only two pathologists took the examination supposedly given by a Civil Service clerk as well as by the Coroner of San Mateo County who was not a physician. The position of Coroner was awarded to Boyd Stephens MD. Acting San Francisco Coroner Ervin Jindrich and forensic pathologist Robert Wright did not take the Civil Service examination. This Civil Service appointment of Boyd Stephens MD as Coroner followed by approval of the San Francisco Board of Supervisors had not included monitoring nor participation by the University of California San Francisco.

During the years 1971-72, Ervin Jindrich MD, acting Coroner, brought innovative ideas to the San Francisco Coroner's Office. In 1972 Boyd G Stephens MD became Coroner, and in 1976 Stephens received his certification in the subspecialty of forensic pathology, making him the first board-certified forensic pathologist to serve as San Francisco Coroner.

After Stephens became Coroner the liaison between the UCSF and the Coroner's Office changed. Stephens, trained as a pathologist, did not require the services of UCSF Pathology Chairman Henry Moon, and Stephens selected his own corps of specialists.

Stephens as Coroner modernized procedures and introduced a standard of quality equal to or better than any medical-examiner or coroner office in the United States. He appeared at most homicide scenes, able to make a pathologist's observations. He took his own photos, directed collection of trace evidence, and cooperated with police investigators to a greater degree than had previous San Francisco Coroners.

Private autopsies were also occasionally performed by Stephens on unusual homicides from counties *outside* San Francisco or in cases wherein the family suspected death was not natural but the deceased's own physician had no basis for reporting the case to a coroner. If there is no obvious cause for a coroner's investigation, the San Francisco Coroner may legally charge a fee for service ($575 per autopsy at the 1980s writing of this history). Usually this extracurricular activity presents no conflict of interest, although in at least one case the Coroner had to pay back the family when autopsy showed that death was in fact accidental and therefore really a Coroner's case. (If a family is to receive double indemnity monies from a life insurance company you realize that their asking for a private autopsy can bring a return much beyond the cost of that autopsy.)

Coroner Boyd Stephens developed the toxicology laboratory in San Francisco in the face of severe budget cuts: to meet costs Stephens used fees from his forensic consultations done outside San Francisco and his fees for private autopsies in non-coroner cases.

As an agent for law-enforcement groups, Coroner Stephens visited jails to examine suspects. He took samples of blood, saliva, and bite-mark impressions, and made other forensic evaluations. Stephens' varied talents proved useful in many ways: he improved x-ray facilities and toxicology, he repaired autopsy saws, and he tightened general procedures in the Coroner's Office.

Stephens brought pathologists whom he selected into the Coroner's Office: first, Norvel (Max) Sisson MD in 1974, and then Jesus Ferrer MD in 1978. At the writing of this history in early 1980s, Stephens' group of experts and consultants included forensic dentist Oliver Harris DDS who assisted in identification of bodies and analyses of bite marks, and forensic anthropologist Roger Hegler PhD who found a never-ending collection of assorted bones from which he determined the age, sex, and even the occupation of the dead. Toxicologists in the Coroner's Office provided increasingly sophisticated analyses for a variety of toxic substances.

Notes to the chapters

Abbreviations for oft-cited references

GCI – *West's Annotated California Codes: Government Code Index.*

SFEB – *San Francisco Daily Evening Bulletin.*

SFMR – *San Francisco Municipal Reports 1850-1930.*

SFMRBB – *San Francisco Municipal Report Blue Book* [continuation of SFMR after 1931 until 1972].

References without specific authors and from calendared sources such as *San Francisco Municipal Reports* are cited on a fiscal-year basis: for example, SFMR 1879 means the 1878-79 fiscal year.

Introduction

1. McGloin pp84-86, 407.

2. SFMR 1880 p381.

3. *Ibid* 1859-1900.

4. SFMR 1867 p266.

5. SFMRBB 1931 p29.

6. Stephens 1979 letter 11 September 1978.

Chapter 1

1. Presley ER pp1-25.

2. GCI 27471, 27472, 27490 pp123-25, 404.

3. Stephens 1982.

Chapter 2

1. Soulé, Gihon, & Nisbet p665.

2. *Ibid,* pp589-91.

3. SFMR 1866 p225.

4. Stewart pp107-29.

5. Lyman 1928 p563.

6. SFEB 1856 15 May.

7. Lyman 1928 pp460-79, Saunders 1956 pp64-68.

8. *Ibid.*

9. *Ibid.*

10. SFEB 1856 14-20 May, Lyman 1928 p478.

11. Lyman 1928 pp463-79, Saunders 1956 pp64-68.

12. Myers.

13. *Ibid.*

14. *Ibid.*

15. Saunders 1960 p214.

Chapter 3

1. SFMR 1865 pp239-43, 1859-1900.

2. Los Angeles Westerners 1956 vol 6 p63.

3. Read & Mathes p123.

4. Kelly p95.

5. SFMR 1869 pp194-212.

6. SFMR 1869-1872.

7. SFMR 1869 p202.

8. *Ibid.*

9. *Ibid* p124.

10. SFMR 1869-1879.

11. *Ibid.*

12. Kelly p95.

13. SFEB 1872 15 March.

14. SFMR 1872 p269.

15. Kelly.

16. Stillman 1967.

17. Lamott pp91-92.

18. SFMR 1872 pp269-272.

19. *Ibid* 1872-4.

20. *Ibid.*

Chapter 4

1. *Western Lancet* 1873.

2. SFEB 1874 20 November.

3. *Ibid.*

4. *Ibid.*

5. SFMR 1873 p399; 1878 p85.

6. Stephens 1980.

7. SFMR 1869 p125.

8. SFEB 1874 24 November front page.

9. SFMR 1883 p20.

10. SFMR 1884 pp211-14.

11. McGloin p166.

Chapter 5

1. SFEB 1875 27 August ff.

2. Lyman 1937.

3. Read & Mathes (for the years 1874-1875).

4. Lyman 1937.

5. SFEB 1875 31 August.

6. *Ibid.*

7. Virchow.

8. Lyman 1937.

Chapter 6

1. Spitz & Fisher p7.

2. SFMR and other municipal records 1859-1980.

3. *American Medical Association Directory* 1906.

4. SFMR 1859-1900 and Duggan 1998
   [phone consultations concerning health statistics].

5. *Ibid.*

6. SFMR 1878 p84.

7. Dorr 1883.

8. Dorr 1881.

9. Dorr 1881a.

10. Dorr 1881b.

11. Soulé, Gihon, & Nisbet pp394-400.

12. SFMR 1881 p120.

13. SFMR 1879-1872.

14. SFMR 1881 p197-98.

15. *Western Lancet* October 1881 p343.

16. SFMR 1859-1900.

17. *American Medical Association Directory* 1934, 1936.

18. SFMR 1882 p43.

19. SFMR 1882 p38.

20. SFMR 1882-83.

21. SFMR 1884 p213.

22. SFMR 1859-1900.

Chapter 7

1. *San Francisco Chronicle* 6 December 1878 article
   quoted in negative campaign publication.

2. *Ibid.*

3. *San Francisco Daily Morning Call* 18 September 1878.

4. SFMR 1866 p235.

5. SFMR 1871 p292-93.

6. SFMR 1893 p336.

7. SFMR 1890-1893.

8. *San Francisco Daily Morning Call* 18 May 1886.

9. Lewis pp51-75.

10. Ibid.

11. *San Francisco Daily Morning Call* 3 November 1909.

Chapter 8

1. SFMR 1890-1901.

2. SFMR 1899 p500.

3. California Academy of Medicine Society Proceedings 1900 pp220-21.

4. SFMR 1902 pp516-32.

5. *San Francisco Chronicle* front page 16 January 1901.

6. SFMR 1915 pp178-79.

7. *Death Reports April-June* 1906 pp516-32.

8. *Book of the Unknown Dead* 1906.

9. *Death Reports* 1906 Book Cii.

10. *Death Reports* 1906 Book C.

11. *Ibid.*

12. *Ibid.*

Chapter 9

1. *San Francisco Chronicle* 2 November 1909 lead article front page.

2. Coroner's Office Statistics 1901-1940.

3. *Ibid.*

4. *Ibid.*

5. *Ibid.*

6. *Ibid.*

7. *Ibid.*

8. *Ibid.*

9. *Ibid.*

10. SFMR 1909 pp884-85.

11. SFMR 1901-1941, Coroner's Office Statistics 1901-1940.

Chapter 10

1. *Survey Report.* 1916. San Francisco: San Francisco City and County.

2. *Ibid.*

3. SFMR 1915-1917.

4. *Survey Report.* 1916. San Francisco: San Francisco City and County.

5. SFMRBB 1958, 1959.

6. *Ibid.*

7. *Ibid.*

8. *Ibid.*

9. Carr 1935 pp274-75.

10. Schultz 1935 pp275-78.

11. Carr 1935 pp274-75.

Chapter 11

1. Turkel 1955, 1953; other material for this chapter learned from colleagues who knew him.

2. Turkel 1955, 1953.

3. Turkel 1953 p1090.

4. Turkel 1953 p1089.

Chapter 12

1. Adler 1967 p97.
2. *Ibid.* 1967.
3. *Ibid.* 1967 pp102, 104.
4. *Ibid.* 1967 p97.
5. CGI 68092, 68095.

Chapter 13

1. Material on Jesse L Carr was collected from varied sources: bibliography from Carr; his son Lawrence Carr Jr MD; author's personal collection of reprints; William Margaretten MD, professor of pathology, University of California San Francisco; and *UCSF Alumni-Faculty Association Bulletin* circa 1967.
2. Carr undated.
3. Carr 1945 pp1-43.
4. Carr & Johnson 1935.
5. Benjamin 1946.
6. Material on Henry D Moon MD was partly collected from Henry D Moon's papers, UCSF Archives.

Chapter 14

1. Material for changes in liaison was collected from Robert Wright MD, Edward Lim, Ervin Jindrich MD, Civil Service documents, and varied personnel preferring to remain anonymous.

References

Sources not here dated

San Francisco Chronicle.

San Francisco Daily Evening Bulletin [SFEB].

San Francisco Daily Morning Call.

Author not available

1878. A Life Record of "Dr" C C O'Donnell: A Fiend's Boast [negative-campaign pamphlet quoting *San Francisco Chronicle*, 6 December 1878].

1873. Our coroner (editorial). *Western Lancet* October 2:614-15.

1881. Editorial. *Western Lancet* October 10:342-44.

1900. California Academy of Medicine Society Proceedings. *Occidental Medical Times* 14:220-21.

1850-1980. *Coroner's Office Statistics.* San Francisco: Archives of the San Francisco Medical Examiner-Coroner's Office.

1906. *American Medical Association Directory.* Chicago: American Medical Association Press.

1906. *Book of the Unknown Dead.* San Francisco: Archives of the San Francisco Medical Examiner-Coroner's Office.

1906. *Death Reports City & County of San Francisco 5 Volumes.* San Francisco: Archives of the San Francisco Medical Examiner-Coroner's Office.

1916. San Francisco City & County Survey Report pp508-45.

1956. *Westerners Brand Book Vol 6.* Los Angeles: Los Angeles Westerners.

Authors' listing

Adler JN. 1967. Coroners' inquests. *University of California Los Angeles Law Review* 15:97-117.

Benjamin H. 1946. A case of fatal air embolism through an unusual sexual act. *Journal of Clinical Psychopathology.* 7:815-20.

Bennett L & Rombo O. Circa 1974 undated. Henry Dukso Moon 1914-1974 [obituary]. San Francisco: University of California San Francisco Archives.

Carr JL & Johnson CM. 1935. Embolism following instrumentation and injection of oil into the urinary bladder. *Journal of the American Medical Association* 104:1973-75.

Carr JL. 1935. The coroner's system. *California and Western Medicine* 43:274-75.

Carr JL. 1945. Status thymico-lymphaticus. *Journal of Pediatrics* 27:1-43.

Carr JL. Undated. My memories of the school of medicine. In *Tales and Traditions* Vol 2 pp148-58.

Dorr LL. 1881. Rabies: a possible cause and a probable preventive. *New York Medical Journal* 34:470-76.

Dorr LL. 1881a. *Un caso de talipes varo-equinae paraltyica. Medicina y Circijia of Central America Guatemala* 2:150-52.

Dorr LL. 1881b. Case of chronic nicotine poisoning and sudden death. *Pacific Medical Medical and Surgical Journal* 23:308-10.

Dorr LL. 1883. Poisoning by belladonna treated by bromide potassium. *Pacific Medical and Surgical Journal San Francisco* 25:58.

Duggan J. 1998. Phone consultation. San Francisco: Public Health Service Vital Statistics.

[GCI] State of California. 1988. *West's Annotated California Codes: Government Code Index.* St Paul: West Publishing [San Francisco: Main Public Library Government Information Center].

Kelly HA. 1912. 1610-1910 *A Cyclopedia of American Medical Biography.* Philadelphia: W B Saunders.

Lamott K. 1961. Chronicles of San Quentin: Biography of a Prison. New York: McKay Company.

Lewis O. 1947. The Phosphorescent Bride—The Case of Dr J Milton Bowers—1885. In *San Francisco Murders,* ed Joseph Henry Jackson. New York: Duell, Sloan & Pearce.

Lyman G. 1928. The sponge. In *Annals of Medical History.* New York: Paul B Hoeber.

Lyman G. 1937. *Ralston's Ring: California Plunders the Comstock Lode.* New York: Charles Scribner's Sons.

McGloin JB. 1978. *San Francisco: The Story of A City.* San Rafael, California: Presidio Press.

Meyers, John 1966. *San Francisco's Reign of Terror.* Garden City, New York: Doubleday.

Presley ER. Circa 1972. *Laws Governing the California Coroner.* Auburn, California 95604: Placer County Sheriff-Coroners [sic] Office, P O Box 69901.

Read JM & Mathes ME. 1958. *History of the San Francisco Medical Society* 1850-1900. San Francisco: San Francisco Medical Society.

San Francisco City and County. 1859-1917. *San Francisco Municipal Reports.* San Francisco: San Francisco City and County.

San Francisco City and County. 1931-1975. *San Francisco Municipal Reports Blue Book.* San Francisco: Municipal Publishing Company.

Saunders J. 1956. California's Fantastic Medical Tradition. In *The Western's Brand Book* Vol 6. Los Angeles: The Los Angeles Corral of The Westerners.

Saunders J. 1960. Data regarding the ashes of Beverly Cole. In *Tales and Traditions*. San Francisco: University of California San Francisco Archives.

Schultz OT. 1935. Why the medical examiner instead of the coroner? *California and Western Medicine* 43:275-78.

[SFEB] *San Francisco Daily Evening Bulletin.*

[SFMR] 1859-1917 *San Francisco Municipal Reports.* San Francisco: San Francisco City and County.

[SFMRBB] 1931-1975 *San Francisco Municipal Reports Blue Book.* San Francisco: Municipal Publishing Company.

Soulé F, Gihon JH, & Nisbet J. 1854. *The Annals of San Francisco.* New York: D Appleton.

Spitz WU & Fisher R. 1980. *Medicolegal Investigation of Death.* Springfield, Illinois: Charles C Thomas.

State of California. 1988. *West's Annotated California Codes: Government Code Index* [GCI]. St Paul: West Publishing [San Francisco: Main Public Library Government Information Center].

State of California. 1998. *West's Annotated California Codes: General Index A to C* pp1312-16. St Paul: West Publishing [San Francisco: Main Public Library Government Information Center].

Stephens BG. 1979. *San Francisco Coroner Annual Report.* San Francisco: San Francisco City and County.

Stephens BG. 1980. Personal communication in San Francisco Coroner's Office.

Stephens BG. 1982. Personal communication in San Francisco Coroner's Office.

Stewart G. 1964. Committee of Vigilance: Revolution in San Francisco 1851. Boston: Houghton Mifflin.

Stillman JDB. 1967. *The Gold Rush Letters of JDB Stillman.* Palo Alto, California: Lewis Osborne.

Turkel HW. 1953. Merits of the present coroner system: statistical comparison with the medical-examiner system. *Journal of the American Medical Association* 158:1086-92.

Turkel HW. 1955. Evaluating a medicolegal office: autopsy index as a comparative standard. *Journal of the American Medical Association* 158:1485-89.

Virchow R. 1896. Postmortem Examinations with Especial Reference to Medico-Legal Practice. Philadelphia: Blakiston, Son & Co.

Index